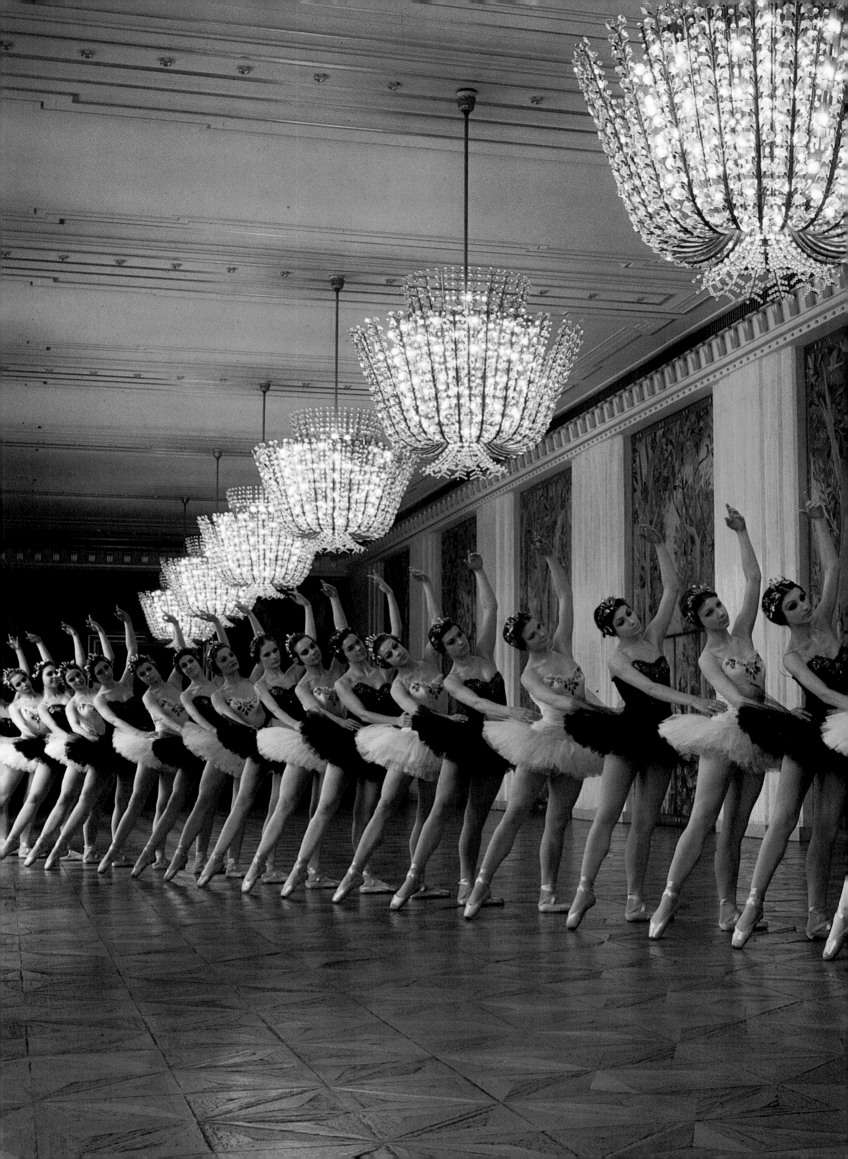

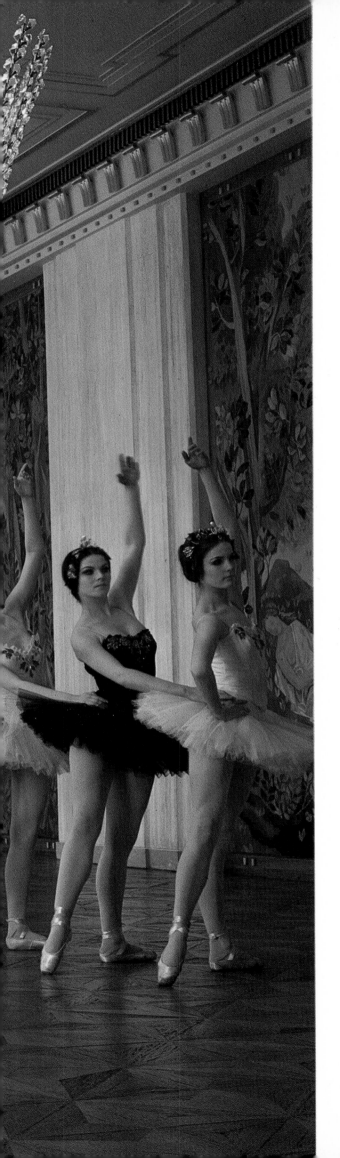

The Magic of
Ballet
by
Catherine Dell

RAND McNALLY & COMPANY

Chicago · New York · San Francisco

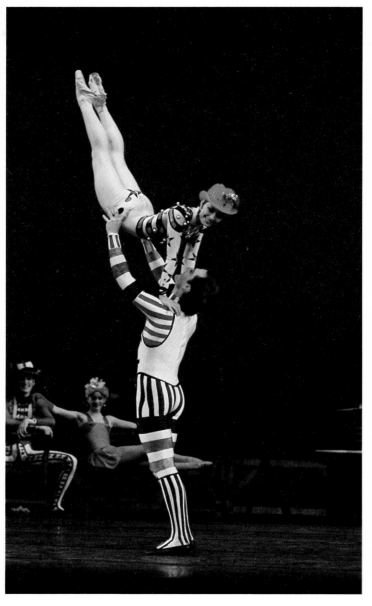

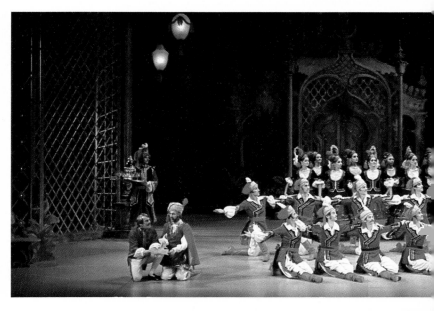

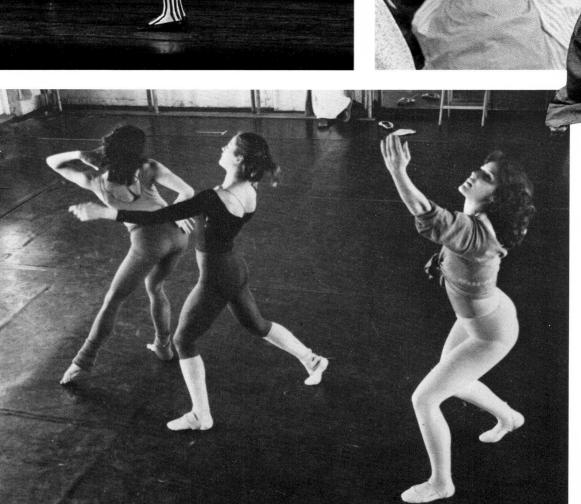

First published in England under the
title Ballet Dancing
© Grisewood and Dempsey Limited 1979
Printed and bound in Italy by
Vallardi Industrie Grafiche s.p.a., Milan

ISBN 528—82262—4
Library of Congress Catalog Card
No. 78—68633

Contents

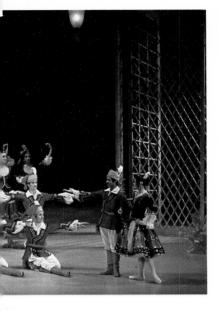

Foreword by
Beryl Grey   9
The Story of Ballet   10
Learning Ballet   15
Ballet Steps   19
Modern Technique   25
The Making of a Ballet   26
A Ballet Dancer's Life   34
Some Great Companies   36
Some Great Ballets   40
Index   45

Cover: Enigma Variations,
*The Royal Ballet's production
with Vyvyan Lorraine and
Robert Mead.*

*Endpapers: The London Festival
Ballet's production of
Swan Lake.*

*Title page: The Vienna State
Opera Company in* Etudes.

*Top left: Desmond Kelly and
Marion Tait in the Royal
Ballet's* Elite Syncopations.
*Top right: The Australian
Ballet's* Merry Widow.
*Bottom: Dancers of the Ballet
Rambert in London in rehearsal.
Bottom right: A scene from
Sir Frederick Ashton's film ballet*
The Tales of Beatrix Potter.
*Below: The Paul Taylor Dance
Company in* Noah's Minstrels.

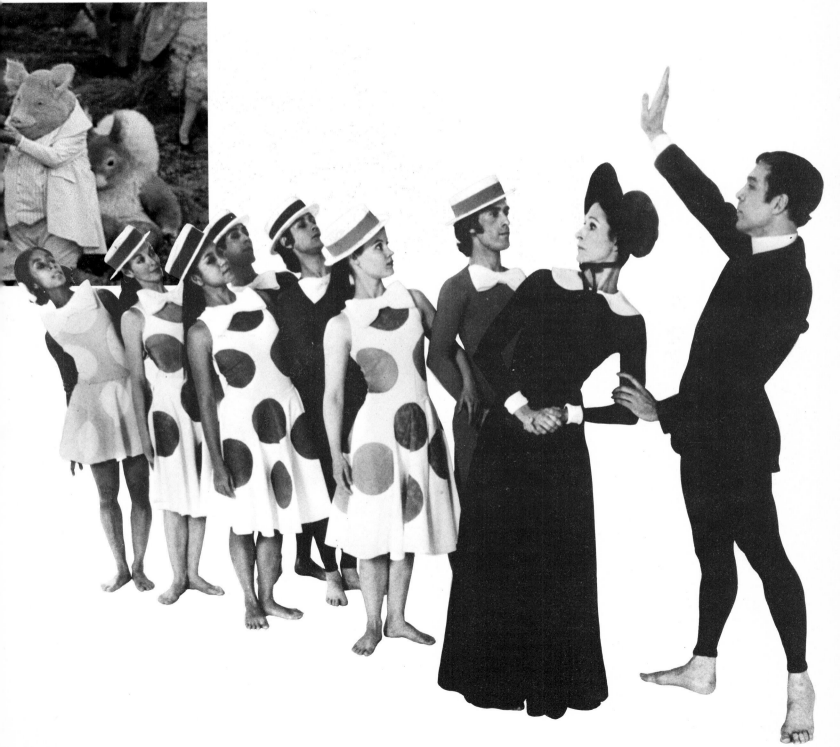

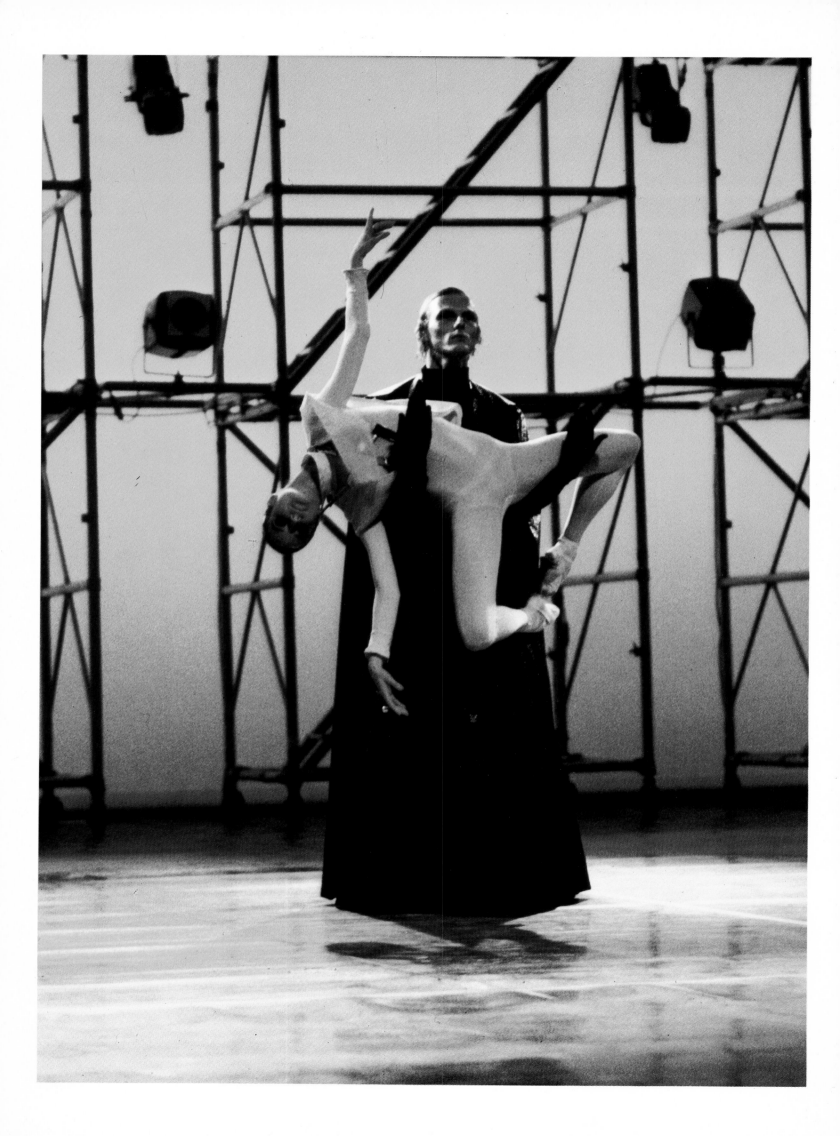

Foreword

When I started my dancing career, ballet was still very much a fledgling art form in England. But since those early days of the then Sadler's Wells Ballet, dance has become one of the most popular forms of entertainment.

During my time as Artistic Director of London Festival Ballet, I have seen audiences grow beyond all recognition. Indeed, one gets spoiled: whereas one would have been thrilled with fifty per cent houses ten years ago, one is disappointed if they fall below eighty or ninety per cent today.

And it is not just in England that this has happened: countries all over the world have developed excellent companies. Nor is the explosion in dance interest confined to classical ballet. Splendid modern dance companies like those of Martha Graham, Erick Hawkins, Murray Louis, Alwin Nikolais, Alvin Ailey, Paul Taylor and Merce Cunningham have fostered their own offshoots so that everywhere dance is flourishing.

What is so encouraging is that there is no longer the rigid differentiation between classical and modern dance that there used to be. There is now a healthy cross-fertilization.

This pattern is now to be found all over the world; wherever one goes one finds enthusiastic audiences, eager to renew acquaintance with a familiar classic as well as developing a growing interest in new works.

This book tells this story clearly and I commend it to you as a first rate introduction to the work that is going on in dance all over the world.

Beryl Grey
Artistic Director of London Festival Ballet

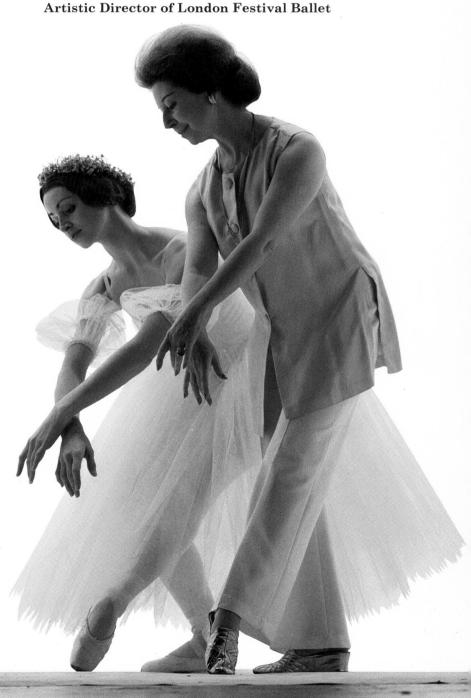

Left: Flemming Flindt, the great Danish dancer and choreographer created the ballet Triumph of Death *for the Royal Danish Ballet to perform first on television and later on stage. Based on Ionesco's* Jeu de Massacre, *the ballet shows how modern man tries to escape from the terrible consequences of the plague. This was one of the ballets introduced into the Danish Ballet's repertoire which was in strong contrast to the tradition of the choreographer Bournonville whose name will forever be linked with that of the Royal Danish Ballet.*

Right: Dame Alicia Markova rehearsing Caroline Humpston for Markova's revival of Fokine's Les Sylphides *for the London Festival Ballet. Dame Alicia Markova was one of the English dancers in Diaghilev's Ballets Russes. She later formed her own company with another English dancer from the Ballets Russes, Anton Dolin. Among her many roles, she had studied* Les Sylphides *with the illustrious Russian dancer and choreographer, Michel Fokine, himself.*

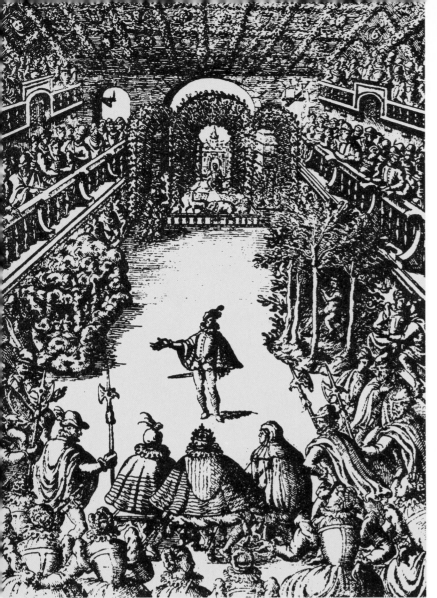

The Story of Ballet

The story of ballet begins five hundred years ago in Italy. In those days, the Italian nobility entertained important visitors with elaborate pageants of poetry, music, mime and dancing. These entertainments, performed by the courtiers, were noted for their lavish costumes and spectacular scenery – often designed by famous artists such as Leonardo da Vinci.

When an Italian, Catherine de Medici, married King Henri II and became Queen of France, she introduced this kind of pageant to the French court. It was a great success. One of Catherine's most dazzling entertainments – and the most famous – was the *Ballet Comique de la Reine* produced in 1581 to celebrate her sister's marriage.

Thanks to Catherine de Medici, ballets – as these festivities were called – became a regular feature of court life in France. They reached their peak of popularity almost a hundred years later under Louis XIV.

The Sun King

Louis XIV, king at the age of five, loved to dance: for twenty years he had daily dancing lessons and first danced in a court ballet when he was only twelve. From then on, he took part in many ballets, usually appearing as a god or some other powerful figure. Louis's title of "Sun King" came from his triumphant role as the sun in the *Ballet de la Nuit*, an extravagant spectacle which lasted over twelve hours. When Louis finally gave up dancing, his courtiers lost interest, too; ballet was taken over by professional dancers and moved from the court to the theatre.

Ballet was now a public entertainment and consisted mainly of singing and dancing. At first, all the dancers were men – they even played female parts – but by the end of the seven-

Above: The Ballet Comique de la Reine, *Paris 1581. This sumptuous entertainment, which took place in the Great Hall of the royal palace, told the story of Circe, an enchantress who turned men into animals. Like all court ballets, it included singing and acting as well as dancing. Court dancing did not involve complicated steps or jumps as the courtiers were restricted by their clothes; instead, it consisted of forming intricate geometrical patterns. With small, delicate steps, the dancers moved in and out, tracing an elaborate sequence of circles, loops, squares and triangles.*

In the Ballet Comique (comique *means dramatic, not funny) the Queen and her ladies took part in the dancing. They were watched by the King and his guests at one end of the hall and by the courtiers in galleries along the sides.*

At one point, the divine messenger, Mercury, descended from a cloud and later, Jupiter appeared in the heavens. These supernatural effects were a regular feature of court ballets, made possible by specially-built machines. In Germany and Italy, even horses appeared in ballets. The Ballet Comique de la Reine *finished at half-past three in the morning; it lasted over five hours, with intervals for refreshments!*

Right: This painting, by the French artist Edgar Degas (1834–1917), shows dancers in a studio at the Paris Opéra. The Opéra was founded by Louis XIV, and is France's main center of ballet. Like most important ballet companies, it has its own school which ranks as the oldest ballet school in the world. Louis founded the Opéra (then called the Académie Royale de Musique) *in 1669; eight years before, he had set up an Academy of Dance. The Academy's first director was the King's dancing master, Pierre Beauchamp. He worked out many of the basic movements in ballet, including the five positions of the feet. Because Beauchamp, a Frenchman, laid the foundations of classical technique and because the world's first ballet school was in France, French became the language of ballet everywhere. In New York, Rome, Sydney, Moscow . . . ballet steps have French names.*

The dancers are wearing the romantic-style costume introduced by Marie Taglioni: a dress with a billowing muslin skirt and a tight-fitting bodice, leaving the neck and shoulders free. In the background, the wooden rail round the wall is called the barre. *All dancers do exercises at the* barre *to warm their muscles before moving into the center for more concentrated practice.*

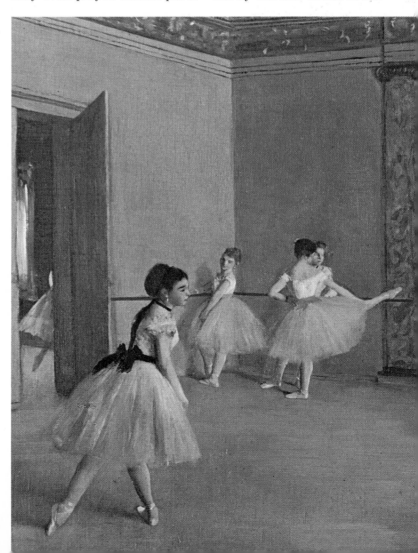

teenth century women were dancing on the stage. One of the most famous dancers was Marie Camargo. She caused a sensation by shortening her skirt and wearing flat shoes so that she could do simple jumps.

In the late 1700s a revolution, led by Jean-Georges Noverre, hit the world of dance. Noverre was a choreographer (a creator of ballets) who believed dancing should be more than meaningless movement: he believed it should tell a story. To help dancers act the story, he did away with singing and the wearing of masks and made them use mime and facial expression. Noverre's ideas totally changed the shape of ballet.

The Romantic Age
The nineteenth century brought more change as balletgoers discovered when they went to the premiere of *La Sylphide* in 1832. Instead of being about classical heroes and heroines, as most ballets were, *La Sylphide* told the tragic story of a beautiful forest sprite who fell in love with a mortal. The performance was like an enchanting dream. It was made even lovelier by the exquisite dancing of Marie Taglioni who played the sprite. She moved across the stage with astonishing grace and lightness and captivated her audience by dancing on *pointe* (on the tips of her toes).

La Sylphide, with its tale of impossible love, its exotic setting and fairy-like heroine, was the first great Romantic ballet. For dancing – like poetry, music and painting – had come under the spell of the Romantic movement which was sweeping Europe. It had exalted emotion, imagination and the supernatural. Another famous Romantic ballet – still popular today – is *Giselle*, a haunting story of dancing spirits.

Ballet moves to Russia
The Romantic period in dancing barely lasted twenty years. When it ended, ballet went into a decline. But not in Russia,

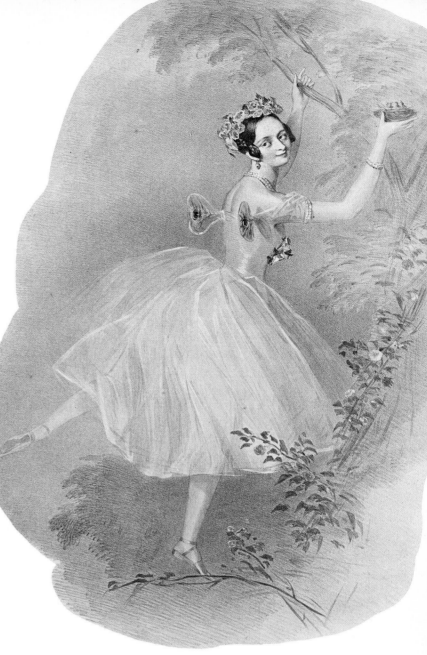

Above: Marie Taglioni moved with amazing lightness. Her father, who trained her and choreographed La Sylphide, once said, "If I heard my daughter dance, I would kill her."

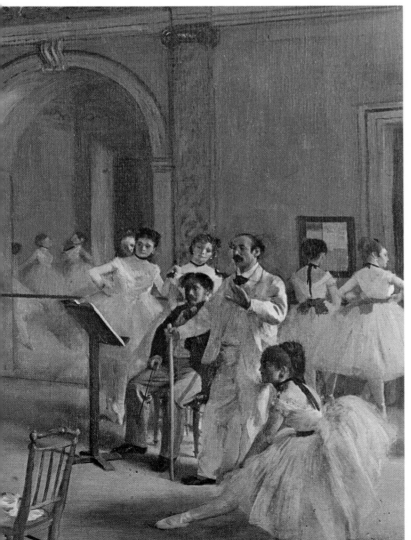

thanks to the Tsar's enthusiastic patronage. The Imperial Ballet companies in Moscow and St. Petersburg, the capital, were renowned for their superb productions and many French dancers and choreographers went to work with them. One Frenchman who made the journey to Russia, in 1847, was the dancer, Marius Petipa. He only intended a short visit but became chief choreographer and stayed for life. Under his influence, the center of the dance world moved from Paris to St. Petersburg (now Leningrad).

During his time in Russia, Petipa choreographed over sixty ballets. They were all long – some had as many as five acts – and they were all designed to show off the great talents of a big company. Each ballet contained important dances for the *corps de ballet* (chorus), brilliant *variations* (solos) for the principal dancers and at least one grand *pas de deux* (duet) for the ballerina and her partner. Petipa always worked closely with both dancers and composers; it was with Tchaikovsky that he created three of the world's best-loved ballets: *Sleeping Beauty*, *Nutcracker* and *Swan Lake*.

Petipa's success did not last for ever. By the end of the century he was considered old-fashioned and, once again, ballet was in a rut. The moment had come for another revolution led, this time, by a Russian, Serge Diaghilev.

11

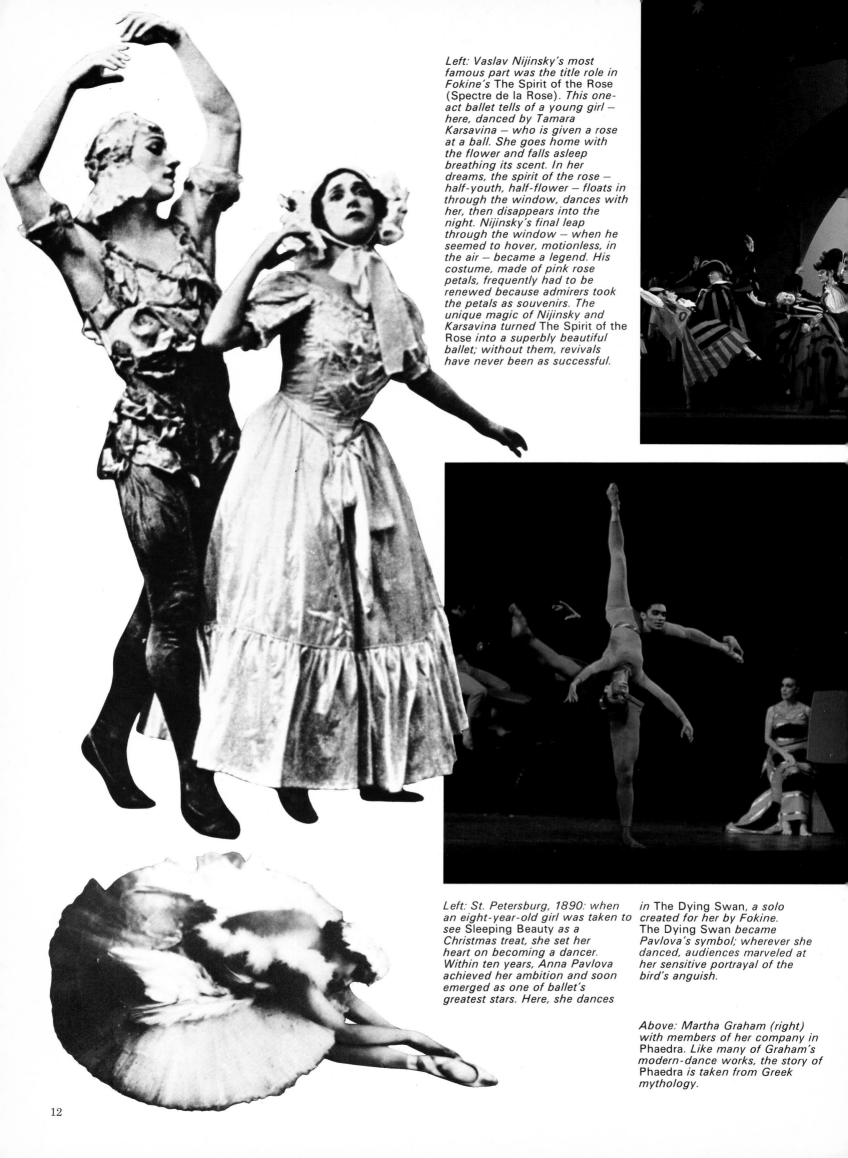

Left: Vaslav Nijinsky's most famous part was the title role in Fokine's The Spirit of the Rose (Spectre de la Rose). *This one-act ballet tells of a young girl — here, danced by Tamara Karsavina — who is given a rose at a ball. She goes home with the flower and falls asleep breathing its scent. In her dreams, the spirit of the rose — half-youth, half-flower — floats in through the window, dances with her, then disappears into the night. Nijinsky's final leap through the window — when he seemed to hover, motionless, in the air — became a legend. His costume, made of pink rose petals, frequently had to be renewed because admirers took the petals as souvenirs. The unique magic of Nijinsky and Karsavina turned* The Spirit of the Rose *into a superbly beautiful ballet; without them, revivals have never been as successful.*

Left: St. Petersburg, 1890: when an eight-year-old girl was taken to see Sleeping Beauty as a Christmas treat, she set her heart on becoming a dancer. Within ten years, Anna Pavlova achieved her ambition and soon emerged as one of ballet's greatest stars. Here, she dances in The Dying Swan, *a solo created for her by Fokine.* The Dying Swan *became Pavlova's symbol; wherever she danced, audiences marveled at her sensitive portrayal of the bird's anguish.*

Above: Martha Graham (right) with members of her company in Phaedra. *Like many of Graham's modern-dance works, the story of* Phaedra *is taken from Greek mythology.*

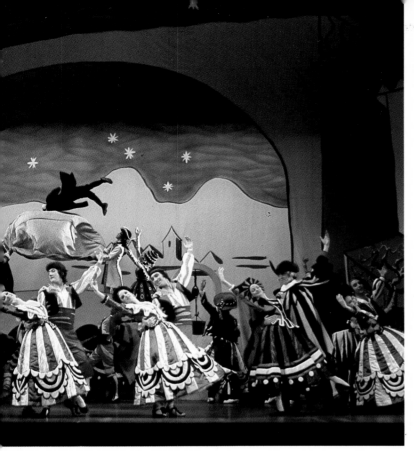

Above: The Three Cornered Hat *was one of the Ballets Russes' many triumphs. During the First World War, Serge Diaghilev, and the company's choreographer, Leonid Massine, took refuge in Spain. While there, they toured the country with the Spanish composer, Manuel de Falla, and a young gypsy dancer. This introduction to Spain inspired Massine to create* The Three Cornered Hat, *a truly Spanish ballet. The action is taken from a story by Pedro de Alarcón; de Falla's music includes folk melodies; Massine's choreography uses traditional dances; while the scenery and costumes designed by Picasso (the famous Spanish artist) provide an authentic atmosphere. This scene from the London Festival Ballet's production is near the end. The hated provincial governor (the wearer of the three-cornered hat) has just been taken away and the villagers celebrate by tossing his effigy in a blanket and dancing a lively jota, a popular Spanish dance. Massine himself revived* The Three Cornered Hat *for the Festival Ballet.*

The Ballets Russes

Serge Diaghilev was a St. Petersburg law student who was not very interested in law. He was much more interested in painting, music, opera, ballet . . . and soon gave up his law studies to edit a new art magazine. Diaghilev and his artistic friends were full of exciting ideas and wanted to try them out, but St. Petersburg was not ready for change. They looked elsewhere and decided on Paris. Diaghilev began by organizing an exhibition of Russian painting in the French capital: it was a great success. Then he treated Paris to Russian music, Russian opera and finally, in 1909, to Russian ballet.

Diaghilev brought his audiences the very best: top dancers from the Imperial companies – among them Anna Pavlova, Tamara Karsavina and Vaslav Nijinsky, and three ballets by the brilliant young choreographer, Michel Fokine.

Parisian balletgoers found Fokine's productions breathtaking. Never before had they seen such superb dancing, such imaginative scenery, such colorful costumes. The Russians were invited back the next year and, in 1911, Diaghilev formed his own company: the Russian Ballet, usually known by its French name, *Les Ballets Russes.* A new era in ballet had begun.

For the next eighteen years – until Diaghilev's death in 1929 – the Ballets Russes delighted audiences in Europe and America. The company owed its enormous popularity to Diaghilev's genius for discovering talent: some of the century's most gifted and creative people worked for the Ballets Russes.

A galaxy of talents

There were the choreographers: Michel Fokine, the rebel who broke with tradition and transformed ballet from a pretty entertainment into a work of art; Nijinsky, dancer and choreographer; Leonid Massine; Nijinsky's sister, Nijinska; lastly, George Balanchine. There were the composers: Stravinsky, Rimsky-Korsakov, Debussy, Ravel, de Falla, Prokofiev: all wrote music for Diaghilev ballets. There were the designers: sets and costumes by Europe's leading artists: Picasso, Utrillo, Matisse, Braque and others. And there were the dancers: Anna Pavlova, one of the greatest-ever ballerinas, who soon left the Ballets Russes to form her own touring group. She spent the rest of her life dancing all over the world, bringing ballet to millions of people. Vaslav Nijinsky was another star dancer; but, after only ten years, insanity ended his dazzling career. Among the other outstanding dancers who worked with the Ballets Russes were Serge Lifar, Olga Spessivtseva, Marie Rambert, Ninette de Valois, Alicia Markova and Anton Dolin.

Diaghilev gave the world a treasury of memorable ballets. Ballets like Fokine's *Les Sylphides, Firebird, Petrushka;* Nijinsky's *L'après-midi d'un faune;* Massine's *The Three Cornered Hat, La Boutique Fantasque;* Balanchine's *The Prodigal Son . . .*

The Ballets Russes scatters

When Diaghilev died the Ballets Russes broke up: its dancers scattered to all parts of the world, taking ballet with them. Serge Lifar went to Paris to become the director, choreographer and principal dancer of the Opéra. Marie Rambert had already gone to London; she was followed by Ninette de Valois, Alicia Markova, Anton Dolin (all three were British, despite their "foreign" stage names). Marie Rambert founded a dancing school and, later, a company which now specializes in modern productions. Ninette de Valois also started a company, the Vic-Wells Ballet, so called because its members (including Markova and Dolin) danced at two theatres, the Old Vic and Sadler's Wells. In time, the Vic-Wells became Britain's Royal Ballet. Diaghilev's last choreographer, George Balanchine, moved to the U.S. where he founded the New York City Ballet. Balanchine brought classical ballet to a country that had pioneered a very different style of dancing: modern dance. Modern dance began with Isadora Duncan, born in San Francisco in 1878. Isadora loved dancing but hated ballet: she found it artificial and stereotyped. Instead, she believed in free spontaneous movement and used to dance barefoot, responding naturally to the music and her feelings.

The new dance

Isadora Duncan's ideas inspired many dancers and choreographers, among them Martha Graham, a fellow American. In the 1930s and 1940s, with Duncan's philosophy as a starting point, Martha Graham developed a new dance system. Her technique, totally different from classical ballet, makes great use of the dancer's back; it also includes twisted, angular body shapes, falls and floor movements. She formed a company to stage her own new-style ballets, set up a school to teach her methods, and stimulated world-wide interest in modern dance. Alwin Nikolais, Merce Cunningham, Glen Tetley and Paul Taylor are only four of the top modern-dance choreographers who have been influenced by Martha Graham's system.

Ballet today

Today's ballet scene is full of variety and contrast. There are long story ballets: many of these, such as *Giselle, Napoli,* and *Swan Lake,* date back to ballet's early days; others, like

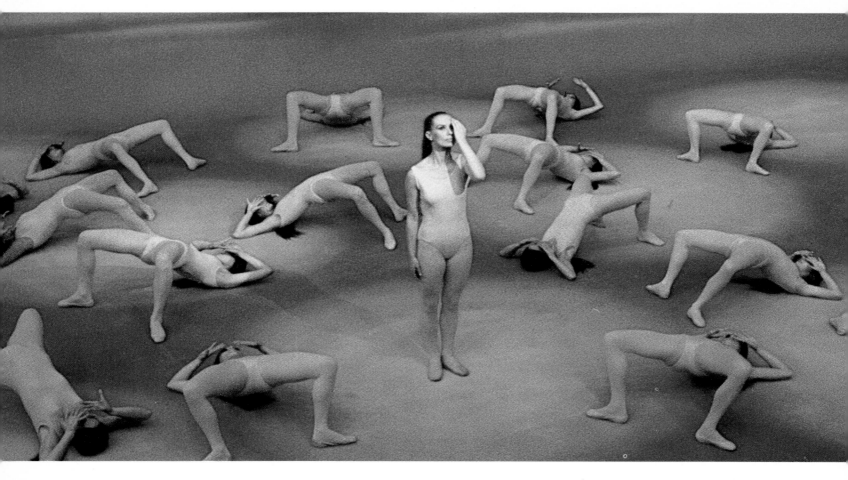

Above: Béjart's company in his version of Sacre du Printemps (Rite of Spring) *– the pagan sacrifice of a young girl. The ballet, created by Nijinsky, caused an uproar at its first night (1913) because it was so unconventional.*

The Taming of the Shrew, *Anastasia* and *Ivan the Terrible* have been created recently. There are also more and more one-act ballets. Some tell a story: two popular examples are *The Dream*, based on Shakespeare's A Midsummer Night's Dream and *Pineapple Poll*, inspired by Gilbert and Sullivan. But a lot of short ballets do not tell a story: they are abstract. Sometimes they describe a mood or an emotion, but basically they are a blend of music and movement. Their appeal and success depends entirely on the choreography.

New themes, new ideas

Of the great modern choreographers, Balanchine, in particular, is famous for his abstract ballets. Mostly they are pure dance works: movement added to music without a trace of time, place or feeling. Among his best-known abstract ballets are *Serenade*, set to Tchaikovsky's Serenade for Strings; *Liebeslieder Walzer*, danced to waltzes by Brahms; *Stars and Stripes*, with Sousa marches; and *Violin Concerto*, performed to Stravinsky's music.

Abstract goes well with modern dance and many modern-dance choreographers concentrate on ballets without stories. They often experiment with revolutionary ideas in sound, lighting, costume and scenery. The results can be sensational: a mixture of new dance rhythms, harsh electronic music, weird noises on tape, blinding spotlights and futuristic props like giant plastic bags, enormous elastic bands, polystyrene blocks. . .

One person who believes in experiment – and on a big scale – is the French choreographer, Maurice Béjart. Béjart and his company, *Le Ballet du XXe Siècle* (Ballet of the Twentieth Century), based in Brussels, put on vast spectacular shows: electrifying mixtures of dance, acrobatics, music, speech, song and striking costumes. Béjart often stages his productions in sports arenas and stadiums; audiences are huge (up to 25,000 people!), young and enthusiastic.

Dance reaches even larger audiences through the movies and television. Many filmed ballets are actual stage productions; some are set up in a studio and photographed there; a few are created especially for the screen, like *The Red Shoes*, starring Robert Helpmann and Moira Shearer, and the Royal Ballet's exquisite *Tales of Beatrix Potter*.

Where to next? In its long history, ballet has moved in many different directions. Because it is alive, it will continue to move. But whatever new dance trends the future brings, there will always be a stage – and an audience – for traditional works. *Giselle*, *Coppélia*, *Nutcracker* are here to stay.

Right: Dancers of the Ballet Rambert in Cruel Garden, *a full-length dance spectacle based on the life and work of the Spanish poet, Garcia Lorca. The Ballet Rambert, Britain's oldest ballet company, is the brainchild of Dame Marie Rambert, one of the most remarkable figures in the dance world. Born in Poland in 1888, Marie Rambert began dancing very young. In 1912, she joined the Ballets Russes to help Nijinsky teach the difficult rhythms of* Sacre du Printemps *and stayed with Diaghilev's group as a teacher and dancer until World War I. She then moved to London and, by 1926, had started her own school and her own company. Today, the Ballet Rambert – consisting of just soloists, no chorus – is known world-wide for its adventurous modern repertoire.*

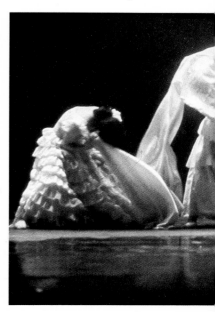

Learning Ballet

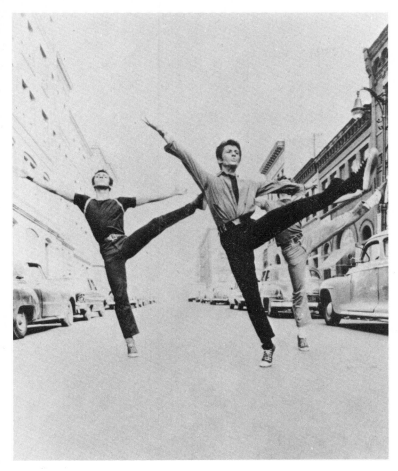

Learning to dance is hard work. It also takes a long time.

From as young as four or five, thousands of girls and boys go to dancing classes. For most of them there is no question of becoming dancers; they have lessons because their parents want them to stand well and move gracefully. Like Alicia Markova: this great British ballerina took up dancing as a cure for flat feet! Sooner or later, however, some of the children show ability and interest and decide to study ballet seriously.

Proper ballet training generally starts at eleven and takes place in a special school. To get into a ballet school, children have to pass an audition and an interview. The audition is taken as a class where the pupils do basic exercises of the kind taught in all dancing schools. The examiners are not watching for clever technique; they are concerned with the candidates' sense of rhythm and their shape: feet, arms, legs, back, knees. Dancing puts a great strain on the body and some types of body stand up to this strain better than others. At the interview, held individually, the examiners are still assessing the child's size and shape; they are also looking for vitality, intelligence and an alert mind.

Musicals on stage and screen often include imaginative dance sequences ranging from the elegant footwork of an old Fred Astaire movie to the fast-moving body rhythms of West Side Story *(above). The exciting dance movements in* West Side Story *were arranged by Jerome Robbins, who also choreographed* The King and I *and* Fiddler on the Roof.

Jerome Robbins, born in New York in 1918, started his ballet career as a dancer. Then, in 1944 (after eight years on the stage), he created his first work, Fancy Free. *This lively ballet, about three sailors on shore leave in New York, was so popular that it was turned into a musical play and a film — with a new title,* On The Town.

In Fancy Free, *and in many of his other ballets, Robbins brings together classical technique and contemporary dance styles. He borrows movements from tap, jazz, folk and discothèque dancing and blends them with formal steps of classical ballet.*

Recognized as America's leading native-born choreographer, Jerome Robbins has composed ballets for several companies, but is chiefly associated with the New York City Ballet. Most of Robbins' recent creations have been presented by them, including his very successful Dances at a Gathering *and* Goldberg Variations, *both abstract, classical works.*

What happens at ballet school?

Ballet school is not all ballet. In many ways it is like any other school. Pupils do ordinary lessons – math, geography, biology, art – and study for the usual high school diploma. And they learn ballet: every day, except Sundays, they have an hour's ballet class. There are other special lessons like music, drama, singing, national dancing (dances from other countries) and history of ballet.

Is such a crowded time-table really necessary? Does a dancer need to know about algebra, amoeba and atmospheric

Below: A junior class at the Stuttgart ballet school. When children join a ballet school at ten or eleven, they have usually had four or five years of dancing lessons. The choice of teacher for these first lessons is vitally important as a bad teacher can do life-long damage in just a few months. Many children with talent have had to give up dancing because their feet and muscles have been ruined by bad training. There are several points to look for in a teacher. What qualifications has he, or she, got? Is he approved by a national dancing association? Do his pupils do well in ballet exams? How many pupils have been accepted by ballet schools?

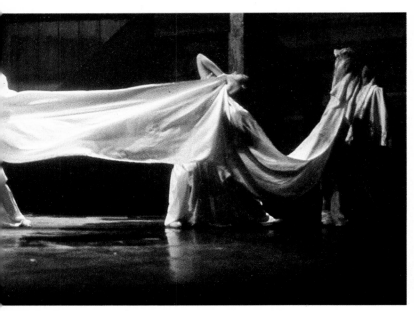

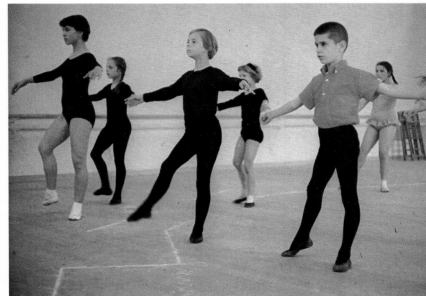

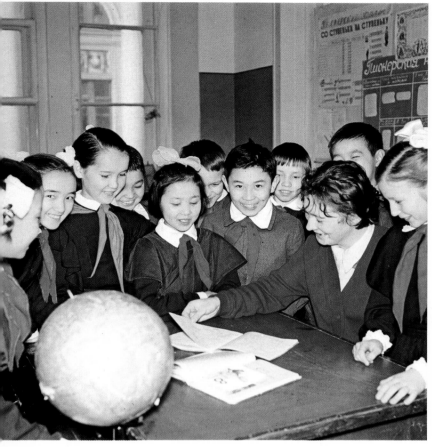

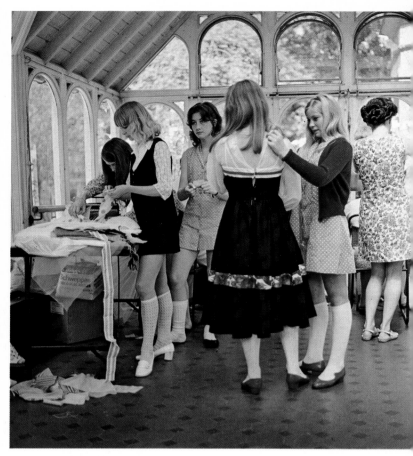

Above: Children, wearing traditional uniform, learn geography at the Kirov ballet school in Leningrad. The school is linked to the magnificent Kirov company (originally Russia's Imperial Ballet) and has trained some of the world's greatest dancers. Among today's ballet stars who studied at the Kirov school and then began dancing with the company are Rudolf Nureyev, Mikhail Baryshnikov and Natalya Makarova.

Above: For the performance staged at the end of term pupils have to learn how to cut, fit and sew costumes.
   Here, girls at the Bush Davies school, London (one of Britain's leading ballet schools), are busy making costumes for their next production. Costumes are always made to measure: they must be an exact fit to allow the dancers to move freely. Whenever possible, costumes are made of lightweight fabrics so that dancers do not feel restricted.

pressure? No, but then very few ballet learners – perhaps only ten in a hundred – actually become dancers. Some give up because they have to: maybe they have grown too large or too tall – a great hefty Romeo or a giant Juliet would look bizarre. Others give up because, by the time they are sixteen, they are no longer as enthusiastic about dancing as they once were: now, they would rather be secretaries, doctors, accountants, nurses . . . The fact that, besides learning to do pirouettes and Polish mazurkas, they have also learned mathematics, English and history makes it possible for them to change direction and go on to other careers. A few put their ballet training to good use, but not as dancers: classes in drama and stage craft are a good stepping-stone for an acting career; controlled, graceful movement is an ideal preparation for modeling. At the end-of-term shows pupils display their new skills. As well as dancing, these shows involve making costumes, painting scenery and wearing stage make-up. Schools attached to major companies sometimes have more exciting opportunities. For instance, when the Royal Danish Ballet put on its most popular production, *Napoli*, children from the company's school form part of the festive crowd in the final act.

A career in ballet
At sixteen, most young people in ballet school have to make an important decision. Should they leave and say goodbye to

ballet or, if they are good enough, stay on for a further two years? The final stage of training is rigorous and only the best of students can survive the pace. There is no longer time for general studies. The whole day (seven or eight hours) is given over to dance: national dancing, historical dancing, tap-dancing, modern stage dancing, Martha Graham-style dance, mime, drama, stage make-up, costumes, choreography, notation, music – and ballet proper. The daily class – still consisting of *barre* work and center practice – now lasts one-and-a-half hours. There are also special sessions for *pas de deux* (dancing with a partner), *tour de force* (advanced steps) and for teaching.

By the time they leave ballet school, students normally have a teacher's certificate and have gained some teaching experience by taking beginners' classes on Saturdays. Some students genuinely want to teach, but for the majority the qualification is a kind of insurance: something to fall back on if they do not succeed as a dancer; something to retire to when their dancing career is over.

In their last year at ballet school, students look for a place with a company. Finding one is not easy: as many as three hundred may audition for just one place! Only a few lucky ones get into top companies; even fewer will ever become top dancers. The five-year-old at dancing class may dream of life as a new Fonteyn or Nureyev; the chances of that dream coming true are remote . . .

WHAT TO WEAR

For dancing, clothing must be simple, comfortable and easily washed. Normally girls (their hair tied well back) dress in short tunics or leotards with cotton socks, when they are very young, and tights, when they are older. Boys wear socks, footless tights and T-shirts.

Everybody, once they start intensive ballet training, uses leg-warmers. These woolly stockings, stretching from the thigh to the calf, may look unromantic, but they are essential — especially at the beginning of class or rehearsal — as they keep the leg muscles warm and flexible.

Shoes are vitally important. At first, children wear flats — soft leather or satin shoes with unblocked (ordinary) toes. When girls are ready to dance on *pointe*, they change over to blocked shoes — shoes with square, solid toes that help them to balance.

Right: Students practicing a folk dance. National dancing is an important part of ballet training as many works feature dances from different countries. In The Nutcracker, *for example, Clara and her prince are delighted by a festival of dances from Spain, Arabia, Turkey, China and Russia; at the Grand Ball in* Swan Lake, *there is an entertainment of Spanish, Neopolitan, Hungarian and Polish dancing; and* The Three-Cornered Hat *includes typical Spanish dances.*

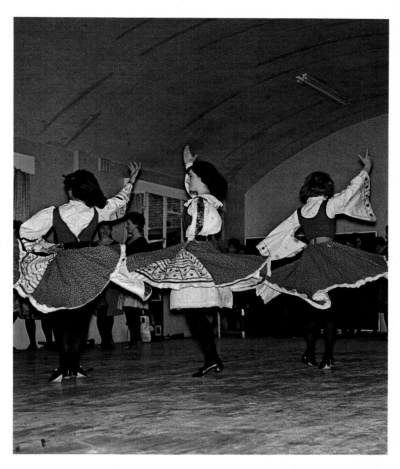

Below: For students at Britain's Royal Ballet school, the highlight of the year is their performance at the Royal Opera House, Covent Garden. Here, Royal Ballet students in Les Patineurs (The Skaters). *Choreographed by Sir Frederick Ashton,* Les Patineurs *is a one-act ballet about a group of young people enjoying themselves on a frozen pond. Despite their lack of experience, they have great fun on the ice. As they happily slip and slide around, they are joined by a youth in blue who dazzles them with skilful turns, leaps and spins. Then, snow begins to fall, the young people glide away and the blue skater is left spinning round.*

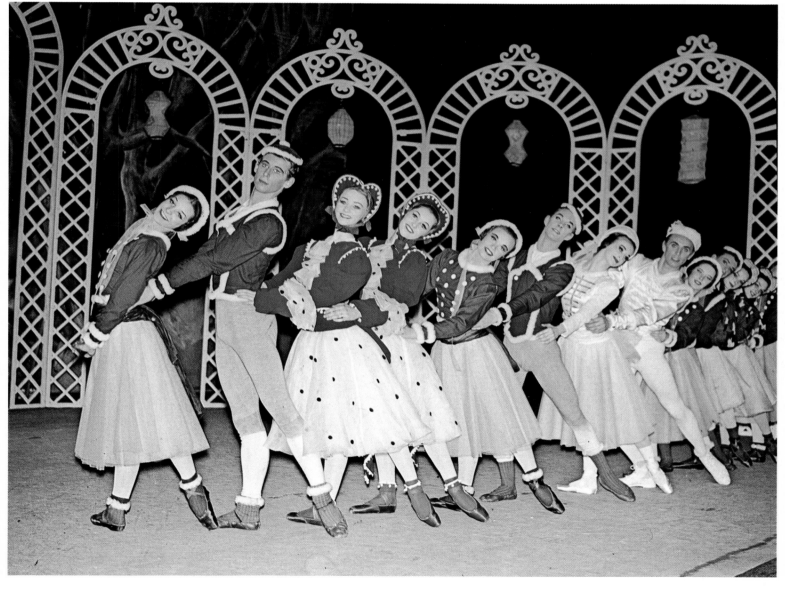

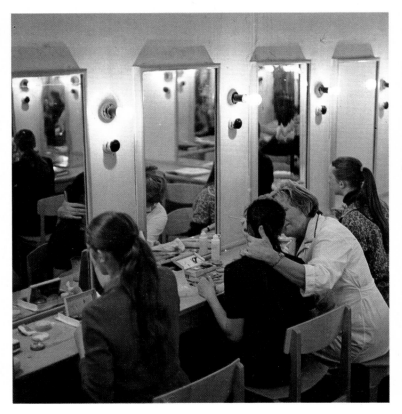

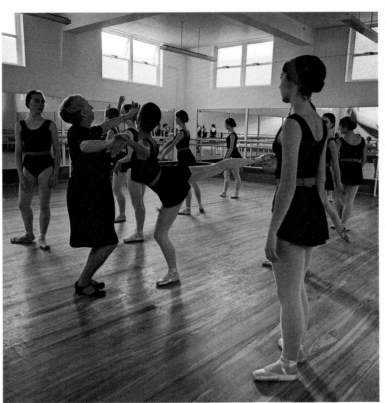

Above: A lesson in stage make-up at Perm choreographic school. Ballet students learn how to put on greasepaint because, in many companies, dancers, even principals, do their own make-up. Perm, an industrial city at the edge of the Ural mountains (USSR), became closely associated with ballet during World War II when the Kirov company was evacuated there from Leningrad. The school, founded in 1945, has produced many gifted young dancers.

Above: Senior students in class. Along the studio wall, behind the barre, is a long, full-length mirror. Mirrors are important: they allow the dancers to watch themselves and so correct any faulty step or position.

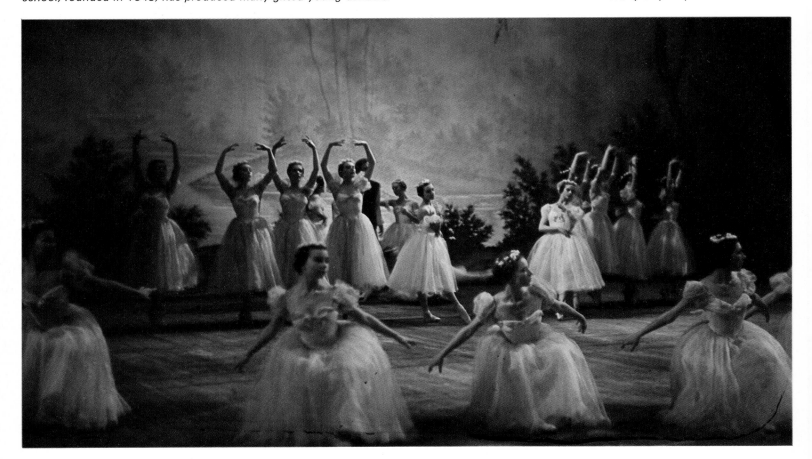

Above: Final-year students from the Bolshoi school in Les Sylphides — a sad, dreamy mood-picture in which a poet dances with ghostly spirits in the moonlit ruins of a monastery. This short, plotless ballet was created by Fokine in 1908 as an examination piece for the Imperial Ballet School in St. Petersburg; it was then called Chopiniana (in honor of its music by Chopin) and is still known by this name in the USSR. In 1909, the Ballets Russes added it to their repertoire, re-named it Les Sylphides and presented it in Paris. Audiences were enchanted — and have been ever since. The Bolshoi school is attached to the great Soviet company. Most of the world's principal ballet companies, such as the Royal Ballet, the Stuttgart Ballet and the Opéra, have their own schools and generally recruit dancers from them, partly because students have been trained in the particular style of the company.

Ballet Steps

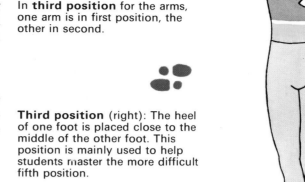

Posture

A dancer must learn to stand correctly. This means standing as tall as possible with the hips directly over the feet, the back straight and all muscles pulled upwards to give the body a slim line.

Turn-out

The placing of the legs is equally important. They should be turned out from the hips down so that the toes point sideways instead of forwards. Turn-out adds beauty to the line of the body and helps the dancer to balance and move easily.

The five positions of the feet

Three hundred years ago, Pierre Beauchamp, Louis XIV's dancing master, first worked out the five positions of the feet; they have changed little since. These positions are fundamental to classical ballet as they are the starting and finishing points for all steps.

The five positions of the arms

Dancing is not just legs and feet. It uses the whole body, especially the arms which must move smoothly, gracefully and expressively. As a foundation for *port de bras* (arm movements) there are five basic positions of the arms. (These vary slightly from one training system to another.) In all five positions, the shoulders are kept down; the elbows are rounded to create a continuous flowing line right through the arm to the finger tips; and the fingers are held freely with the thumb pulled gently towards the palm.

In **third position** for the arms, one arm is in first position, the other in second.

Third position (right): The heel of one foot is placed close to the middle of the other foot. This position is mainly used to help students master the more difficult fifth position.

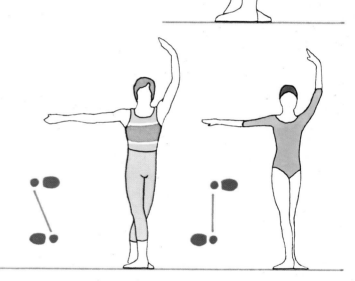

Fourth position (above): There are two fourth positions. The fourth *ouverte* (French open) is the easier: The feet are parallel, a step apart, with the heel of the forward foot in line with the heel of the back foot. The fourth *croisée* (crossed) is harder: the heel of the forward foot is in line with the toe of the back foot.

In **fourth position** for the arms, one arm remains in second position; the other, with slightly bent elbow, is raised over the head, but not too far back.

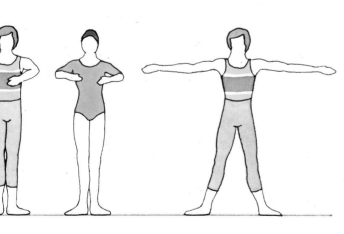

First position (above): The heels are together and both feet are completely turned out to form a single straight line.

The arms are in **first position**: raised in front of the body and delicately curved. The palms of the hands face inwards, the fingers almost touch.

Second position (above): The turned-out feet are still in a straight line, but the heels are about 12 in (30 cm) apart.

The arms, sloping gently from the shoulders, are opened to the sides in **second position**. Again, they are slightly curved; elbows, wrists and hands are held up so that the line is not broken. The palms face outwards.

Fifth position (right): The feet are crossed so that they lie flat beside each other, with the toe of one behind the heel of the other.

Both arms are held over the head in **fifth position**. The palms face inwards and fingers are close, but not touching.

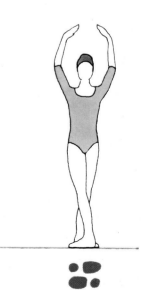

At the barre

Classwork always begins at the *barre* – a wooden rail fixed to the wall at waist height. The dancer holds the *barre* lightly (never leans on it) and does a series of exercises to warm the body, loosen the joints and make the muscles strong and supple. Some of these exercises are shown here.

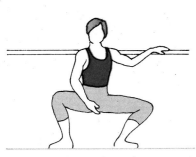 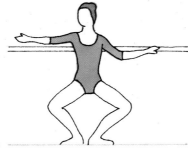

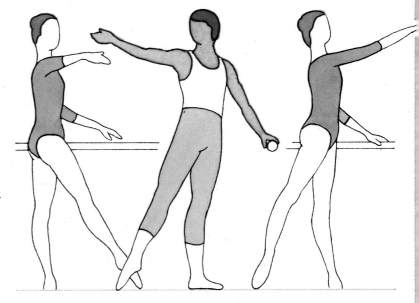

Pliés (above): *Plié* comes from the French verb *plier*, to bend. Every class starts with this slow bending exercise which relaxes the leg muscles, helps turn-out and develops flexibility of the knees. In a *plié* the knees are bent, in line with the turned-out feet, until the thighs are parallel with the floor. *Pliés* are done in all five positions: in the closed positions (first, third and fifth) the heels are raised; in the open

positions, the heels remain on the ground. The illustration shows a *plié* in second position.

Demi-pliés: *Demi* means half and a *demi-plié* is exactly what it says: a half-*plié*. The knees are only slightly bent and the heels never leave the ground – not even in the closed positions. *Demi-plié* acts as a preparation for many steps including jumps and pirouettes. Here, a *demi-plié* in first position.

Battements tendus (above): *Battements* (beating movements) form part of several exercises. In a *battement tendu* the leg, well turned-out, is extended to the front, side and back without lifting the toes from the floor. The main aim of the exercise is to stretch the foot; *tendu* comes from the verb *tendre*, to stretch.

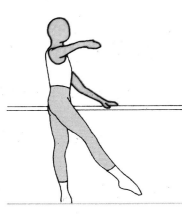 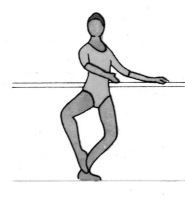 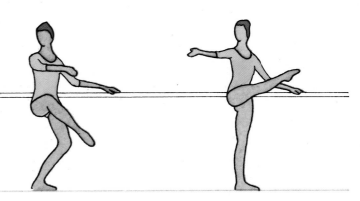

Battements tendus jetés (or *glissés*) (above): *Jeté* means thrown; *glissé*, means slide and *battement tendu jeté* is similar to the *battement tendu* but the foot is lifted off the ground very slightly. It is done more quickly than the *battement tendu* and gives lightness to the legs.

Battements fondus (above and right): *Fondre* is to melt and the *battement fondu* is a smooth, floating movement. In the starting position the working foot is placed just above the supporting ankle, on the *cou de pied* (the 'neck' of the foot); the working leg is then extended to the front, side and back; the supporting knee is bent at the beginning, but straightens as the working leg stretches out. This exercise is important as it is used for preparing jumps.

Right: Anthony Dowell, a principal with the Royal Ballet and one of Britain's leading dancers. Even the most experienced artists must practice every day and, like every other dancer, they have to begin with exercises at the barre.

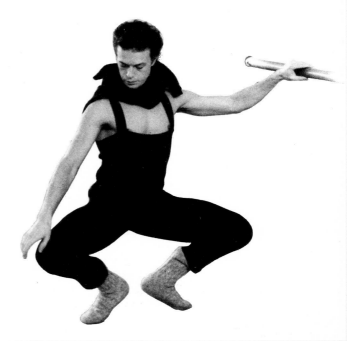

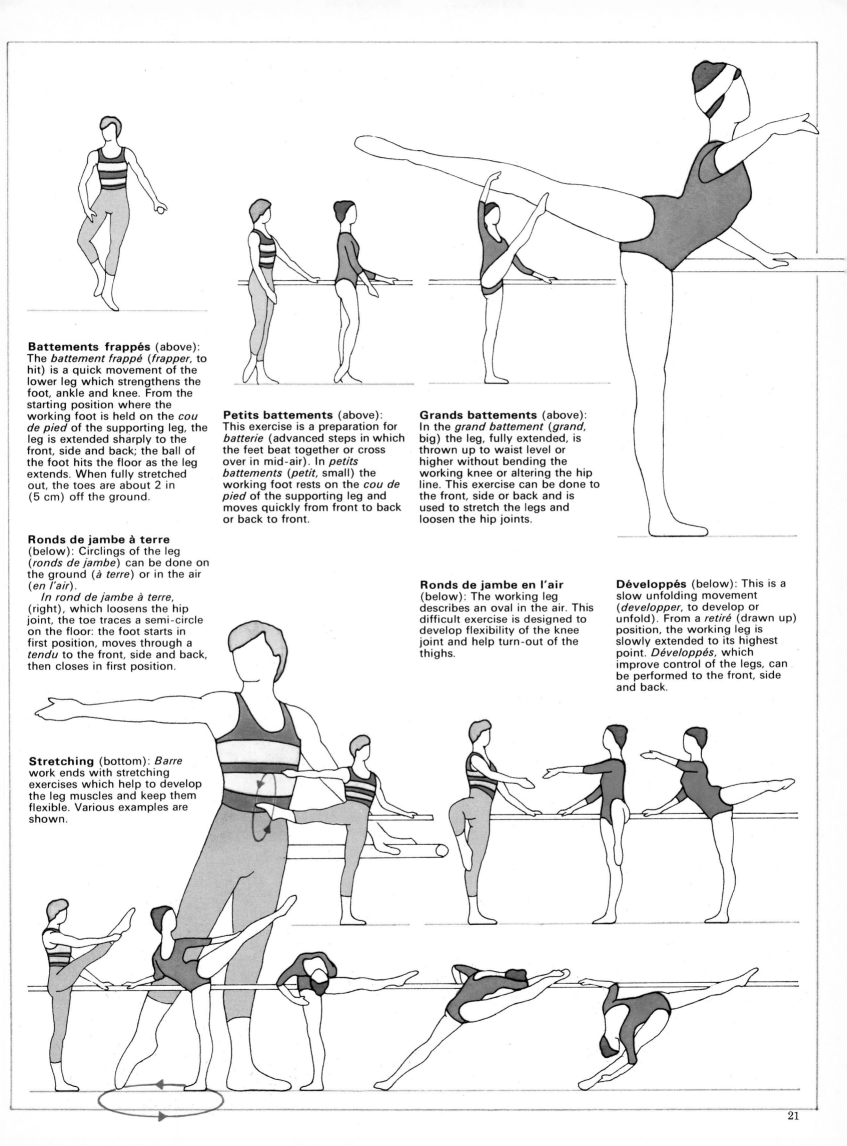

Battements frappés (above): The *battement frappé* (*frapper*, to hit) is a quick movement of the lower leg which strengthens the foot, ankle and knee. From the starting position where the working foot is held on the *cou de pied* of the supporting leg, the leg is extended sharply to the front, side and back; the ball of the foot hits the floor as the leg extends. When fully stretched out, the toes are about 2 in (5 cm) off the ground.

Ronds de jambe à terre (below): Circlings of the leg (*ronds de jambe*) can be done on the ground (*à terre*) or in the air (*en l'air*).

In rond de jambe à terre, (right), which loosens the hip joint, the toe traces a semi-circle on the floor: the foot starts in first position, moves through a *tendu* to the front, side and back, then closes in first position.

Petits battements (above): This exercise is a preparation for *batterie* (advanced steps in which the feet beat together or cross over in mid-air). In *petits battements* (*petit*, small) the working foot rests on the *cou de pied* of the supporting leg and moves quickly from front to back or back to front.

Grands battements (above): In the *grand battement* (*grand*, big) the leg, fully extended, is thrown up to waist level or higher without bending the working knee or altering the hip line. This exercise can be done to the front, side or back and is used to stretch the legs and loosen the hip joints.

Ronds de jambe en l'air (below): The working leg describes an oval in the air. This difficult exercise is designed to develop flexibility of the knee joint and help turn-out of the thighs.

Développés (below): This is a slow unfolding movement (*developper*, to develop or unfold). From a *retiré* (drawn up) position, the working leg is slowly extended to its highest point. *Développés*, which improve control of the legs, can be performed to the front, side and back.

Stretching (bottom): *Barre* work ends with stretching exercises which help to develop the leg muscles and keep them flexible. Various examples are shown.

Classwork: center practice

After half an hour at the *barre*, the muscles are warmed and ready for more concentrated work. This takes place in the middle of the studio and is called center practice. For beginners, center practice mostly consists of repeating *barre* exercises without the *barre*. But as the months go by, there is less repetition and more time is spent on *port de bras*, pirouettes, poses, *adage* and *allegro*. *Adage*, (from *adagio* an Italian musical term meaning slowly) is used in ballet to describe a slow dance. *Adage* work in class is a sequence of slow exercises which aid controlled movement and balance. In contrast, *allegro* means quick and lively and includes fast turning and jumping steps and *batterie*. Some of the work done in center practice is shown here and on the next page.

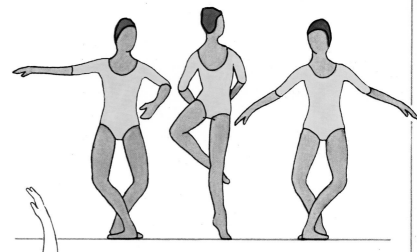

Pirouettes (above): The pirouette (*pirouetter*, to whirl) is a complete turn done on one leg. There are many different kinds of pirouettes. One of the most common begins with a *demi-plié* in fourth position *croisée* and ends with a *demi-plié* in fifth position; during the turn, the working foot is drawn up with the toes just below the front of the supporting knee. The illustration shows a pirouette *en demi-pointe*.

Arabesques (above): The *arabesque* is a pose in which the dancer stands on one leg with the other leg raised to the back. There are various kinds of *arabesque* as the arm positions differ and the supporting leg can be bent or straight. The body is always held upright except in the *arabesque allongée*, when it is parallel to the floor, and in the *arabesque penchée* when it slopes downwards. The illustration shows a first *arabesque*.

Attitudes (left): The *attitude* is a pose based on a famous statue of Mercury. In the basic position, the dancer stands on one leg with the other leg, bent at the knee, lifted behind. The corresponding arm is raised above the head and the other is extended to the side. There are various versions of this pose. The illustration shows an *attitude croisée* (crossed) in which the raised leg is bent behind the supporting leg.

Echappés (below): *Echappé*, which literally means escaped, is a simple jumping step. The dancer starts with a *demi-plié* in fifth position, springs into the air, opens the feet and ends with a *demi-plié* in either second or fourth position.

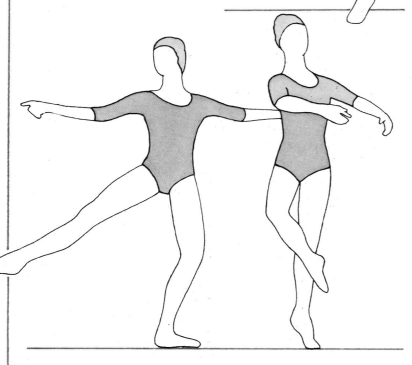

Fouettés (left): *Fouetté* (*fouetter*, to whip) is a fast turning step. The working leg whips out to the side and back into the knee as the dancer turns on the supporting leg. *Fouettés* are usually performed in a series: the most famous sequence occurs in *Swan Lake* where Odile does thirty-two.

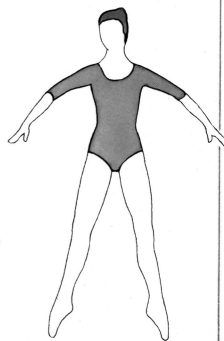

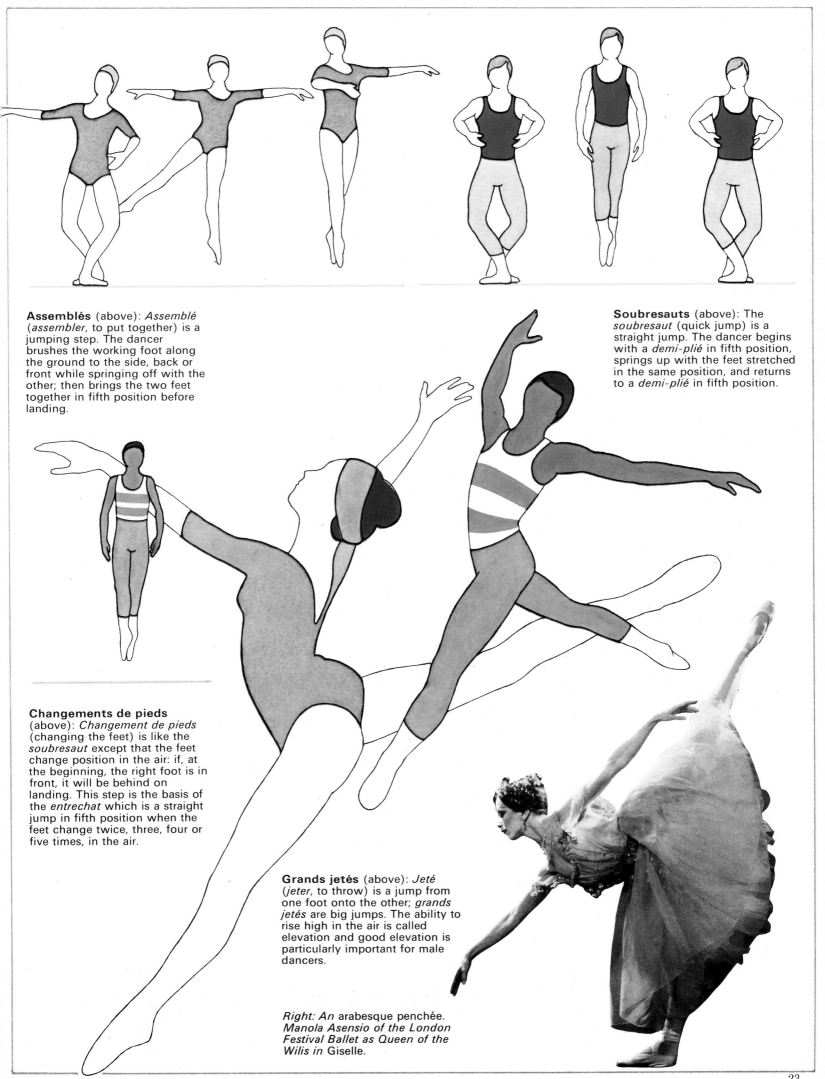

Assemblés (above): *Assemblé* (*assembler*, to put together) is a jumping step. The dancer brushes the working foot along the ground to the side, back or front while springing off with the other; then brings the two feet together in fifth position before landing.

Soubresauts (above): The *soubresaut* (quick jump) is a straight jump. The dancer begins with a *demi-plié* in fifth position, springs up with the feet stretched in the same position, and returns to a *demi-plié* in fifth position.

Changements de pieds (above): *Changement de pieds* (changing the feet) is like the *soubresaut* except that the feet change position in the air: if, at the beginning, the right foot is in front, it will be behind on landing. This step is the basis of the *entrechat* which is a straight jump in fifth position when the feet change twice, three, four or five times, in the air.

Grands jetés (above): *Jeté* (*jeter*, to throw) is a jump from one foot onto the other; *grands jetés* are big jumps. The ability to rise high in the air is called elevation and good elevation is particularly important for male dancers.

Right: An arabesque penchée. *Manola Asensio of the London Festival Ballet as Queen of the Wilis in* Giselle.

Classwork: on pointe and pas de deux

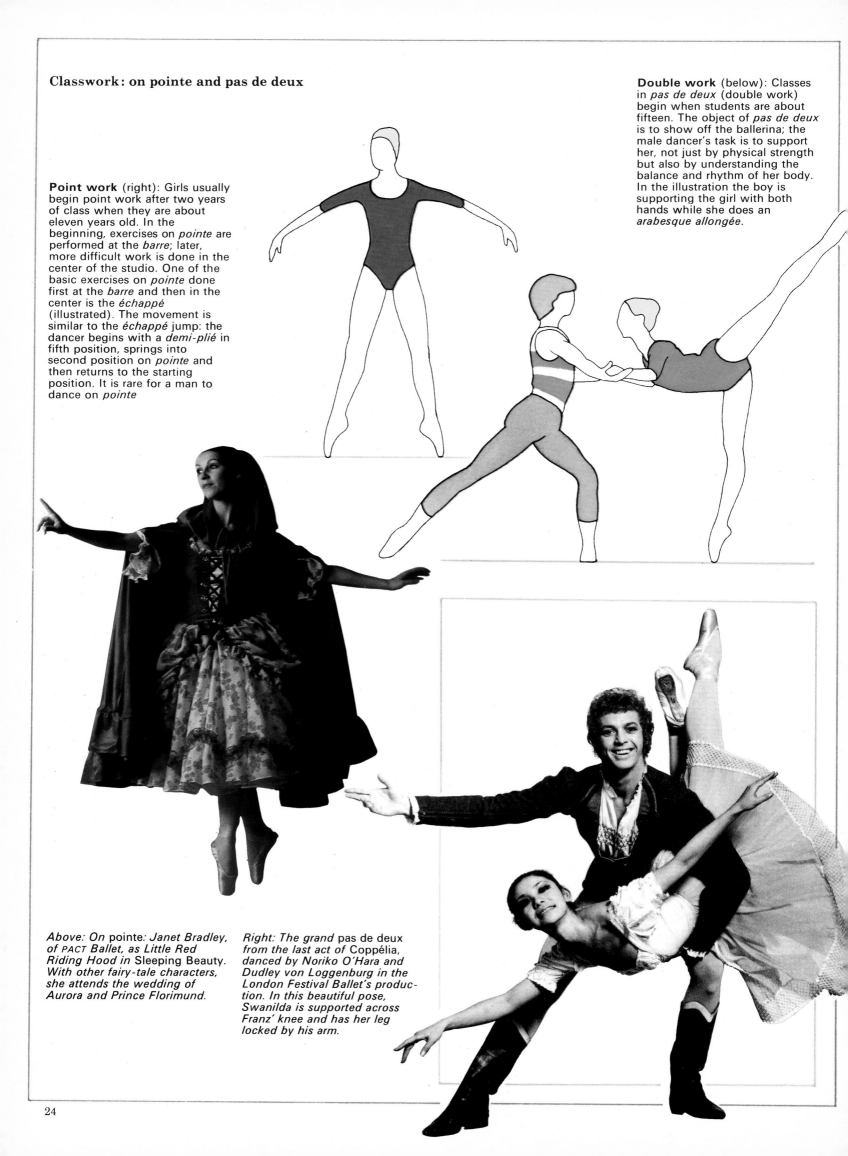

Point work (right): Girls usually begin point work after two years of class when they are about eleven years old. In the beginning, exercises on *pointe* are performed at the *barre*; later, more difficult work is done in the center of the studio. One of the basic exercises on *pointe* done first at the *barre* and then in the center is the *échappé* (illustrated). The movement is similar to the *échappé* jump: the dancer begins with a *demi-plié* in fifth position, springs into second position on *pointe* and then returns to the starting position. It is rare for a man to dance on *pointe*

Double work (below): Classes in *pas de deux* (double work) begin when students are about fifteen. The object of *pas de deux* is to show off the ballerina; the male dancer's task is to support her, not just by physical strength but also by understanding the balance and rhythm of her body. In the illustration the boy is supporting the girl with both hands while she does an *arabesque allongée*.

Above: On pointe*: Janet Bradley, of* PACT *Ballet, as Little Red Riding Hood in* Sleeping Beauty. *With other fairy-tale characters, she attends the wedding of Aurora and Prince Florimund.*

Right: The grand pas de deux *from the last act of* Coppélia, *danced by Noriko O'Hara and Dudley von Loggenburg in the London Festival Ballet's production. In this beautiful pose, Swanilda is supported across Franz' knee and has her leg locked by his arm.*

24

Modern Technique

Students at ordinary ballet schools – studying classical technique – often learn a few modern dance movements during their final year. But students who want to concentrate on modern dance go to special schools. As modern dance is constantly evolving, several different systems exist: the most popular is the Martha Graham technique.

At Graham schools, class is divided into three parts. The first part consists of floor work. The floor serves the same purpose as the *barre* – it aids balance. On the floor, the student performs a series of standard exercises in various sitting, kneeling and lying positions. These exercises prepare the dancer's back and arms for the remainder of the class.

After floor work comes center practice – exercises, done standing, that mostly involve the Graham technique's basic principle: the back as the source of movement from "contraction and release" and the "spiral". Breathing is the origin of contraction and release: breathing out (contraction) makes the back and shoulders curve, breathing in (release) makes the back straighten. The spiral is the foundation of all turns: hips, waist, shoulders and head turn – or spiral – round the spine.

The third section of class includes traveling steps, sequences across the floor, jumps and falls.

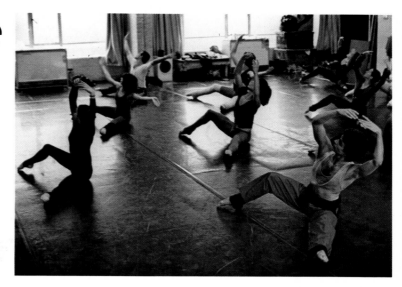

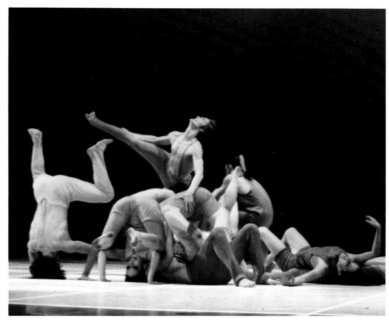

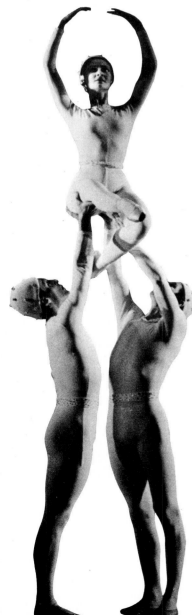

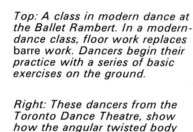

Top: A class in modern dance at the Ballet Rambert. In a modern-dance class, floor work replaces barre work. Dancers begin their practice with a series of basic exercises on the ground.

Right: These dancers from the Toronto Dance Theatre, show how the angular twisted body shapes used in modern dance are completely different from the graceful flowing lines of classical ballet.

Left: Members of the Royal Ballet in Sir Frederick Ashton's Monotones II. The strange sexless costumes, white tights, leotards and caps, might well belong to a modern dance work. In fact, Monotones II is purely classical. This brief ballet, for just three dancers, consists of graceful, unhurried movements and beautiful poses that resemble sculpture.

Right: The Nikolais Dance Theatre in Tensile Involvement. Alwin Nikolais, an American choreographer, designer and composer, believes in "total" theatre: all parts of a production are equally important. To make sure his company's presentations are as "total" as possible, Nikolais creates the entire work himself. He invents the movements, composes the music, designs the scenery, props and costumes, and arranges the lighting. Often, his props, like the elastic cords here, become an extension of the dancer and so form unexpected and unearthly shapes. His work is also famous for its spectacular use of color and light.

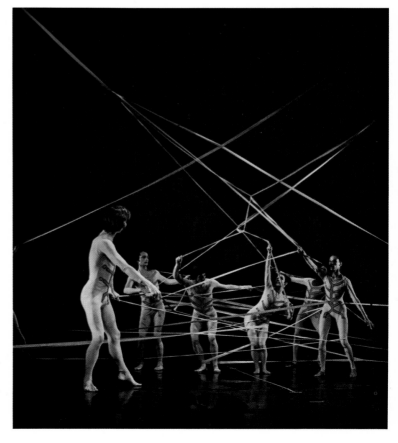

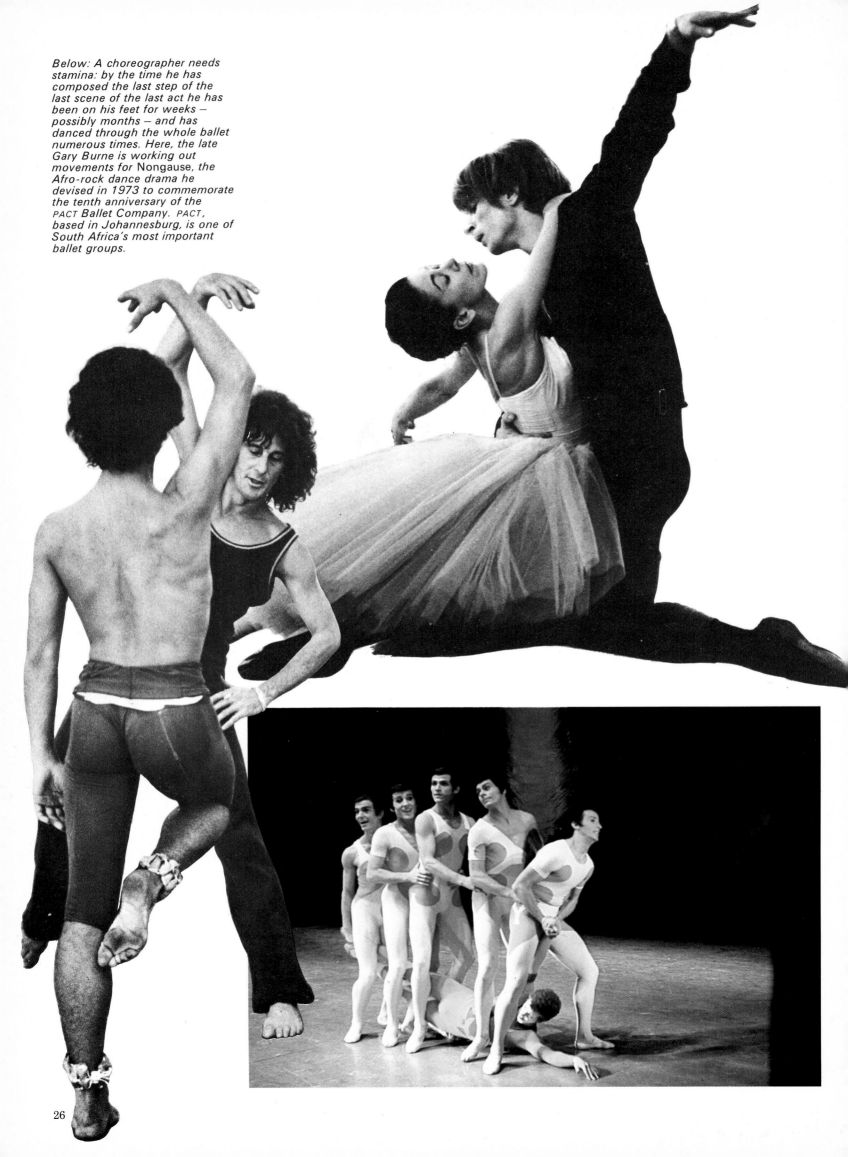

Below: A choreographer needs stamina: by the time he has composed the last step of the last scene of the last act he has been on his feet for weeks — possibly months — and has danced through the whole ballet numerous times. Here, the late Gary Burne is working out movements for Nongause, the Afro-rock dance drama he devised in 1973 to commemorate the tenth anniversary of the PACT Ballet Company. PACT, based in Johannesburg, is one of South Africa's most important ballet groups.

The Making of a Ballet

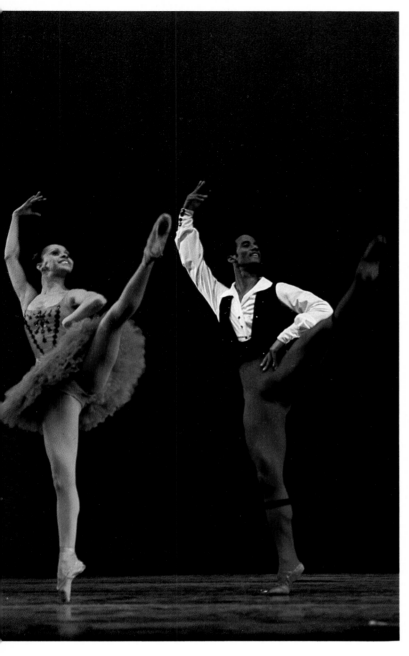

The choreographer is the mastermind behind a ballet. He decides on the story or theme, selects the music, chooses the designer and arranges the steps and dance movements: hence the name choreographer (dance composer) from the Greek *choreos*, dance, and *grapho*, to record.

The starting point, the original idea, can be almost anything. Ballets have been inspired by the Bible (*Prodigal Son*), Chinese shadow-boxing (*Embrace Tiger and Return to Mountain*), a famous Rembrandt painting (*The Anatomy Lesson*), Southern spirituals (*Revelations*), a game of chess (*Checkmate*), one of La Fontaine's fables (*Two Pigeons*), the bicentennial (*Union Jack*), Scott Joplin's ragtime music (*Elite Syncopations*) . . . in fact, by all kinds of stories, music, events, moods and emotions.

All ballet stories, however unalike they may be, have one thing in common: simplicity. As there are no words, everything has to be indicated through movement. If the plot is too involved the dancing becomes complicated and the audience confused. Situations which normally rely on words have to be avoided. How does a character explain, without speaking, that she is the hero's first cousin or that he is thirty-six years old?

Once a choreographer has settled on an idea, he develops it into a scenario, dividing the action into scenes and acts. One, two or three acts? How many scenes to an act? What to put into each scene? With the scenario as a basic framework, the choreographer can begin his unique task of creating the dances.

The choreographer at work

When composing a ballet, the choreographer is probably doing several things: he may be using traditional steps and sequences, arranging existing steps in an unusual way and originating totally new movements. As a result, most ballets are a mixture of convention and invention, of the expected and the unexpected.

Choreographers have different methods of working. Some concentrate on first getting the feel of the ballet – music, theme, characters; they then work out the precise steps with the dancers in rehearsal. Others study the music phrase by phrase, arrange each dance movement accordingly and go to the first rehearsal with the whole ballet planned in detail. Marius Petipa, the Frenchman who went to Russia and gave the world *Sleeping Beauty*, *Nutcracker* and *Swan Lake*, liked to prepare dance patterns beforehand. He had a set of little figures, like chess pieces, which he used to place on the table in various positions. When a particular grouping pleased him, he would note it for future use. In contrast, George Balanchine, the contemporary Russian-American choreographer, does little advance work except for listening to the music over and over again and choosing his cast. He thinks out actual movements when he is alongside the dancers in the rehearsal studio.

Before turning to choreography, both Petipa and Balanchine were dancers and this is true of most choreographers. Having had dancing experience, they can fully appreciate a dancer's reactions and abilities; they also know which steps are possible and which are not.

Above left: Often, the outstanding skill of a dancer motivates a choreographer to create a ballet. Sir Frederick Ashton, for instance, has always been inspired by Margot Fonteyn's brilliant talents and has composed several ballets for her. In Ondine *(1958) — the story of a water sprite who falls in love with a mortal — Ashton gave Fonteyn one of her most exquisite roles. He set the seal on the superb partnership of Margot Fonteyn and Rudolf Nureyev by creating* Marguerite and Armand *(1963). This short ballet, based on Alexandre Dumas' novel,* The Lady of the Camellias, *tells of the tragic love-story of Armand and the dying Marguerite in a series of passionate and tender flashbacks.*

Left: A game of poker provided the starting point for one of George Balanchine's ballets, Card Game (Jeu de Cartes), *set to music composed by Stravinsky. Here members of the Stuttgart Ballet dance a new version arranged by their late director, John Cranko.*

Above: Literature is a popular source of inspiration for choreographers and many novels, poems and plays have been transformed into ballets. Don Quixote *is no exception: in 1869, Petipa choreographed a four-act version of the Spanish classic; almost a hundred years later, Balanchine produced a totally new presentation of Cervantes' masterpiece. Even more recently Karel Shook, co-director of the Harlem Dance Theatre (the world's only black classical company) arranged the* pas de deux *from Balanchine's version for the group's repertoire. Here, the* Don Quixote Pas de Deux *is danced by Joseph Wyatt and Elena Carter, of the Harlem company.*

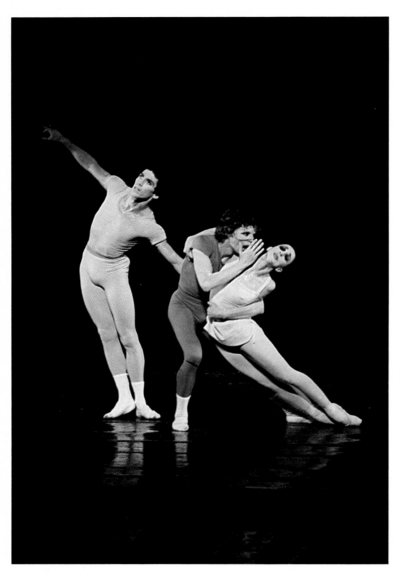

Music is a basic ingredient of ballet. Sometimes, it even provides the initial inspiration: a particular melody captures the choreographer's imagination and moves him to create a ballet. Many great choreographers have at times worked in this way. George Balanchine used Tchaikovsky's Serenade for Strings as a starting point for his ballet *Serenade*; John Cranko studied two of Bach's Brandenburg Concertos and then choreographed *Brandenburg 2 and 4*; Frederick Ashton, inspired by Elgar's music created a ballet about the composer and his friends, *Enigma Variations*.

In other cases, the idea comes first, the music second: the choreographer decides on the story or theme, then thinks about an accompaniment. He may ask a composer to write some music especially for that ballet, as Petipa asked Tchaikovsky to compose scores for *Sleeping Beauty*, *Swan Lake* and *Nutcracker*. From the choreographer's point of view, specially-composed music is ideal. He can specify its length, its pace and its mood and so be certain that music and dance really do harmonize. But such scores are expensive, so choreographers often have to work with existing music.

What music? From Bach to Pop

Since ballet began, an enormous variety of music has been used: concertos, symphonies, folk, opera, jazz, pop, electronic, Gilbert and Sullivan . . . A choreographer generally tries to avoid a well-known melody because the public will have already given it their own meaning and may have difficulty in accepting a new interpretation. Inevitably, existing music is not always a perfect fit: parts may be too quick, too slow, too long or too short for what the choreographer has in mind. Then the music has to be arranged – perhaps by the orchestra conductor, perhaps by a composer – to suit the dance sequences.

Choreographers use their music in different ways. For some, the main purpose of music is to produce background atmosphere and they do not link it with the dancing; others totally synchronize movement and music; while others make the choreography relate to the music without insisting that each step match each beat. Occasionally, choreographers introduce voices into their productions. For example, *Song of the Earth* has two singers and there is a narrator in *Peter and the Wolf*. A few choreographers are even experimenting with music-free ballets, with the dancers performing in absolute silence.

Above: Inspired by the music and words of Mahler's Das Lied von der Erde, *Kenneth MacMillan created* Song of the Earth – *possibly his finest work – for the Stuttgart Ballet.* Song of the Earth, *about death as an inevitable part of life, has three main figures: the masked messenger of death, a man and a woman. The messenger claims the man, then returns, with the man, for the woman. Here, the Stuttgart company's top dancers, Marcia Haydée, Egon Madsen (messenger) and Richard Cragun in* Song of the Earth.

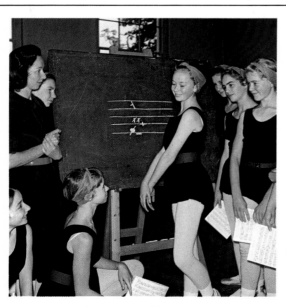

Above: Joan Benesh teaching notation to pupils of the Royal Ballet School.

PUTTING IT ON PAPER

Ever since ballet began, people have been trying to write it down. A system of written dance, based on letter abbreviations for certain steps, was used as long ago as 1460. Over the years, other methods using signs and symbols appeared. None was really successful.

For nearly five centuries, in fact, there was no satisfactory means of recording dance. As a result, many great ballets were lost for ever; others survived by being passed on from one generation of dancers to another. This century, however, saw the introduction of two efficient systems of notation (the noting down of dance). One was developed by Rudolf von Laban (1879–1958), the other by Rudolf Benesh (1916–1975). Labnotation is widely used by modern dance groups, while the Benesh system, more suited to classical ballet, has been adopted by many companies.

The sample of Benesh below is from *Rite of Spring*.

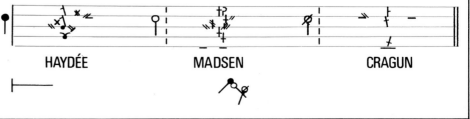

HAYDÉE   MADSEN   CRAGUN

The ballet in rehearsal

A ballet comes alive in rehearsal. No longer is it just an idea in the choreographer's head – or jottings in his notebook.

At rehearsals, the dancers themselves help create the ballet. This is particularly true if the choreographer is one of those who arrives in the studio with an overall view of what the dancing is about but with no detailed plan for each movement. Then the choreographer and the dancers construct the ballet together. The choreographer listens to a few bars of the music, thinks up some steps, tries them out, then makes the dancer copy his movements. Perhaps part of the sequence seems wrong: the choreographer discusses it with the dancer, suggests a different movement, goes through it himself, watches the dancer try it, alters a step slightly, watches the dancer again. Finally, the choreographer feels the movements are right. He moves on to the next musical phrase and the next dance sequence. Even if the choreographer does decide all the steps in advance, when he gets to rehearsal and starts working with the dancers, he invariably finds himself changing and adapting his original ideas.

Creating ballet is slow work: it can take an hour of rehearsal to produce one minute of dance. For a full-length ballet, the choreographer starts working with the principals a year or more before the production opens. Six months later, rehearsals become more concentrated and the principals, soloists and chorus work together. Much nearer the first night there are rehearsals on stage: some in costume, some with the orchestra. And all with the choreographer who does not hesitate to make last-minute changes in position, timing, gestures, facial expression – even steps.

Top right: One of the world's greatest-ever choreographers, Russian-born George Balanchine, trying out a step with a dancer from his own company, the New York City Ballet. Balanchine is a very musical choreographer: he believes music is basic to ballet and when creating a new work he immerses himself in the score.

Below right: Sir Frederick Ashton rehearsing members of the Royal Ballet in Lament of the Waves. *The choreographer constructs the whole ballet: as well as arranging the steps, he decides when the dancers move, where they move to, which way they face, what gestures they make, whether they look happy, sad, afraid . . .*

Below: Class at the Ballet Rambert. Dancers always begin their working day with class. This routine practice keeps their muscles strong and supple and prepares them for rehearsal – which can last several hours !

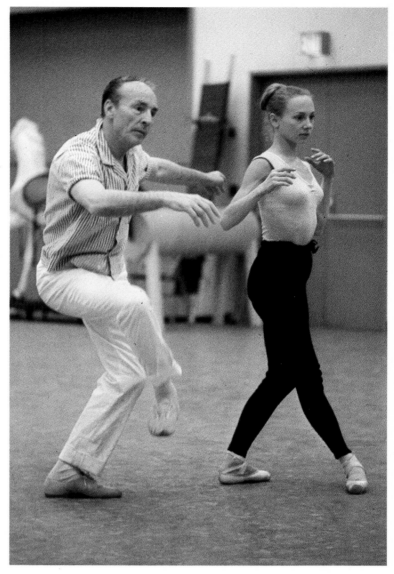

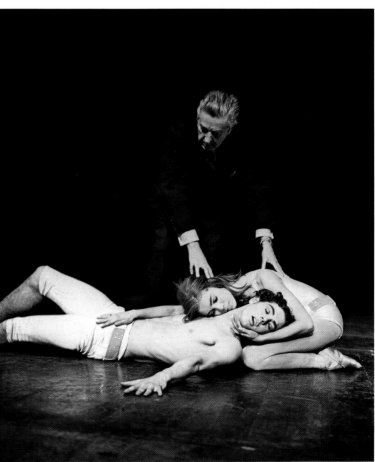

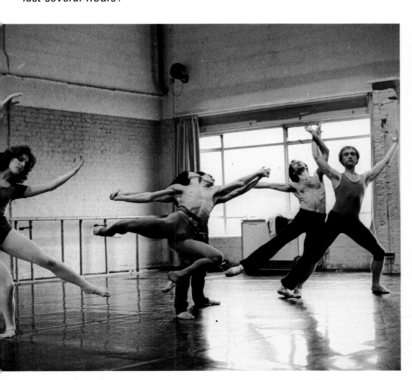

29

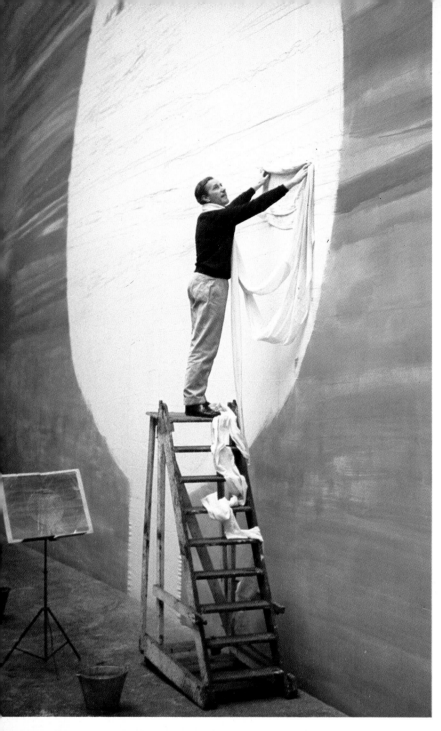

Building another world

As soon as the choreographer's ideas begin to take shape, he calls in a designer. Designers are artists and their job is to create a stage picture, using scenery and costumes, to match the theme of the ballet.

The designer starts work about a year before the ballet has its debut. He discusses the project with the choreographer, and puts his own thoughts down on paper: maybe rough sketches on the backs of old envelopes, maybe elaborate plans. More discussion, more drawing until, at last, the choreographer feels the design captures the right atmosphere – and leaves enough room for dancing.

Most full-length story ballets need a lot of scenery. Before any of it is made a scale model of the set is built on a miniature stage. Detailed plans are drawn up from the model and used to construct the real scenery.

Many ballet companies have their own workshops: there, wood, plastic, metal and fabric are shaped into castles, forest glades, town squares . . . While the workshop is noisy with saws and hammers, brushes are busy in the paint shop where the backcloth, a huge canvas some 22 yards long and 13 yards high, hangs against one wall. With great sweeps of color, artists transform it into a country garden, a city street, a mountain valley . . .

Pigeons and pumpkins

On a smaller scale, there are props to prepare: items like a horse for Kate and Petruchio in *The Taming of the Shrew*, swords for Romeo and Juliet's warring families, the old toymaker's key in *Coppélia*, a bicycle for one of Elgar's friends in *Enigma Variations*, Cinderella's pumpkin coach, even live birds for *The Two Pigeons*. And there are special effects to plan: the Sylphide's escape up James' chimney, the magic transformation of the Nutcracker into a Prince . . .

Modern one-act ballets tend to use scenery and props sparingly: partly to concentrate attention on the dancing itself and partly to save money. In Glen Tetley's *Pierrot Lunaire*, for example, the stage is bare except for a scaffolding tower; the set for Sir Frederick Ashton's *Symphonic Variations* consists of a simple green backcloth, nothing more; while vague cloud formations are the only stage decoration in Jerome Robbins' *Dances at a Gathering*. In ballets where there is little scenery, lighting often plays an important part. Changes in color, in brightness and in range can convey mood and atmosphere just as forcibly as painted canvas and wood do in traditional productions.

Designers work not only on new ballets, but also on new productions. *Swan Lake* has delighted audiences for nearly ninety years. All these audiences have heard the same Tchaikovsky music, but they have not all seen the same dancing, the same scenery, the same costumes. For, in the course of its ninety years, there have been as many as thirty major versions of *Swan Lake*: each version with its own choreography and its own design.

Above: Sydney Nolan, the Australian artist, designed the costumes and scenery for the Royal Ballet's production of Rite of Spring. *He is seen here painting the backcloth.* Rite of Spring, *a new version by Kenneth MacMillan of* Sacre du Printemps, *tells how a primitive tribe offers a young girl in sacrifice to the god of spring; the victim is forced to dance herself to death.*

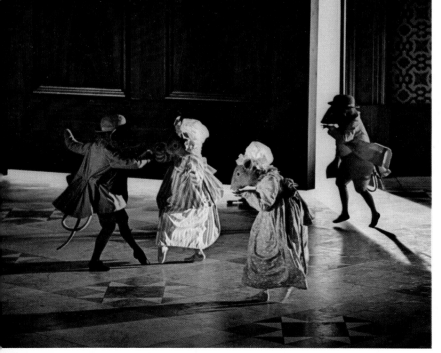

Left: Created especially for the cinema, The Tales of Beatrix Potter *was choreographed by Sir Frederick Ashton and danced by members of the Royal Ballet. It was a real challenge for the designer. Much of the scenery was built larger-than-life to make the performers appear tiny. Here, in the Mouse Waltz, the enormous tiles reduce the dancers to mice-size. Each animal head was modeled individually. The mask-maker worked from Beatrix Potter's drawings and from life: for Hunca Munca (a mouse), he had a real mouse in his studio.*

BEHIND THE SCENES

At a ballet performance, attention is focused on the dancers. To a lesser extent, the audience is aware of the orchestra and front-of-house staff: the box office staff, the usherettes and program-sellers. But there are many people involved in that performance whom the public never sees.

Firstly, the three originators: choreographer, composer and designer. Then, those who transform the inspiration into reality: the scenic builders and artists who make the scenery; the stage hands who move the scenery on and off stage; the tailors and cutters who make the costumes; the wardrobe staff who wash and iron between performances; the wig-master who dresses the wigs; the make-up artists who create the face of a witch or simpleton or fairy queen or clown; the props department who can supply anything from a donkey to a dagger; the electricians who light up the scene — or darken it; the administrators who fit the ballet into the company's schedule and advertise it; and the stage manager who, on the night, co-ordinates it all . . .

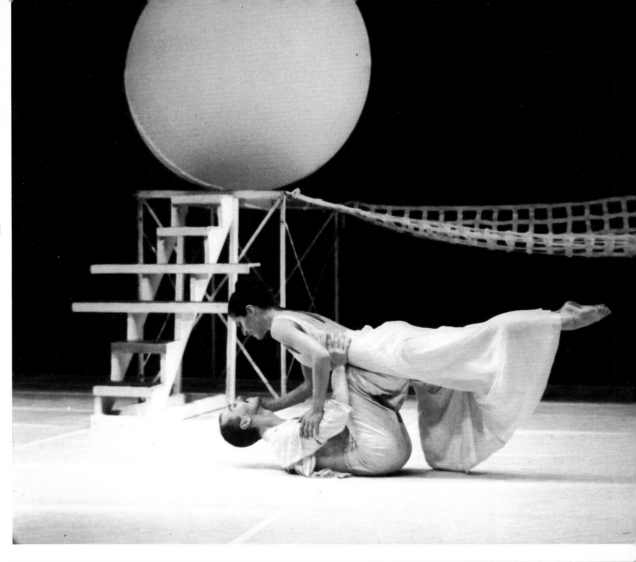

Top: Members of the Toronto Dance Theatre in Delicate Balance. *The symbolic arrangement behind the performers is very basic. Limited scenery and props are used in many abstract works. What little is used is invariably simple and often multi-purpose. A collection of metal ladders, for instance, can be grouped to form a tower or a house or a cage or a prison. A length of white sheeting, worn as a cloak over the shoulders, becomes a shroud when wound round the body and looks like a baby if it is rolled up and cradled in the arms.*

Right: The opening scene of La Fille Mal Gardée: *as dawn breaks over Widow Simone's farmyard, the cockerel and hens wake up and greet the new day with a perky dance. Like most story ballets, this production (by the National Ballet of Canada) makes full use of scenery and costume to create the right setting and atmosphere. This company has British origins. After a triumphant tour of North America in 1949 by the Sadler's Wells Ballet, an English dancer and choreographer, Celia Franca, set up a company in Toronto. The company is now directed by Alexander Grant, formerly of the Royal Ballet.*

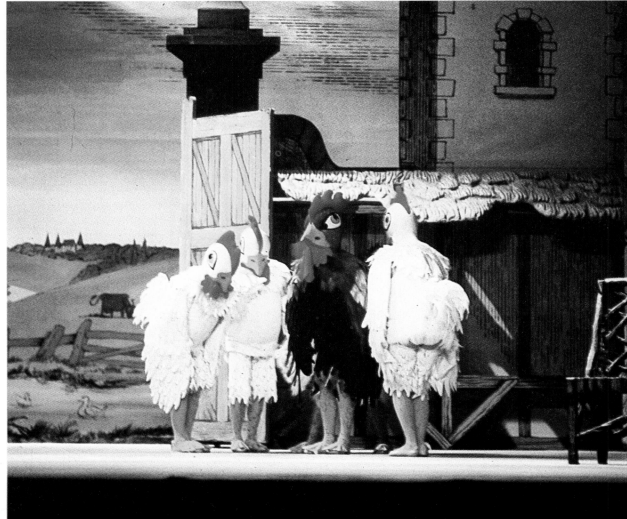

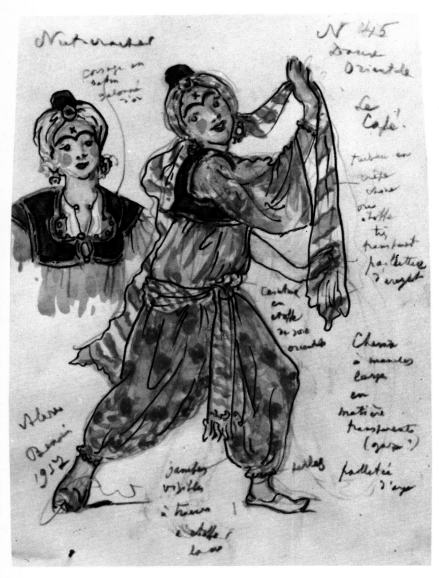

Dressing up for the part

Costumes are an essential part of design. In a story ballet, they help create character: a kilt for James in *La Sylphide*, sailors' vests for the crew of *Hot Cross Bun* in *Pineapple Poll*, a rich velvet doublet for Romeo, plain cotton smocks for the peasants in *Giselle* . . . In an abstract ballet, they are used to project mood and theme. For Serge Lifar's pure dance work, *Noir et Blanc* (Black and White), the costumes mirror the title: girls wear white tutus, while men dress in white shirts and either black or white tights. Balanchine's plotless ballet, *Jewels*, is inspired by emeralds, rubies and diamonds; accordingly, the costumes are green, deep crimson and dazzling white.

If the ballet is set in a distinct historical period such as Ancient Rome (*Spartacus*) or in a precise country like Spain (*Three Cornered Hat*), the designer begins by finding out about Roman or Spanish costumes, then develops his own ideas and makes some rough sketches. These are discussed with the choreographer and the wardrobe (the department responsible for making costumes) and, when everybody is in agreement, clear detailed drawings are prepared.

Making the costumes

The moment has now come to choose the fabrics. All kinds of material are used: velvet, satin, cheesecloth, leather, silk, synthetic fibres . . . And net for tutus. Since it is frequently impossible to find the right material in the right shade, fabrics often have to be dyed. Dyeing also guarantees a perfect color match between parts of a costume made in different materials (such as nylon tights and cotton tunics) and between costumes and scenery: in abstract ballets, the dancers' clothing often harmonizes with the backcloth.

Each costume is made individually – it must be a perfect fit if the dancer is to move properly – and much of the sewing is done by hand. So it is hardly surprising that a full-length ballet, which may require as many as three hundred costumes, means two or three hectic months' work for the wardrobe. As well as dresses, skirts, trousers and shirts, there are many accessories like hats, wigs, shoes, jewelery and gloves. Generally these are not made by the wardrobe but by theatrical suppliers.

However elaborate they look, costumes must be as light as possible yet extremely hard-wearing. Light to allow free and effortless dancing; hard-wearing to survive hours of athletic movement and constant cleaning because, by the end of a performance, clothes are soaked in sweat and many items have to be washed every day.

Not all productions give the wardrobe so much work. Many of today's abstract ballets are performed in practice clothes. Balanchine, for instance, regularly ignores costume: in his *Agon* and *Violin Concerto*, the dancers are dressed simply in tights and leotards or T-shirts.

Below: During their crowded day, dancers often have to take time off from rehearsal for a costume fitting in the wardrobe. Here, a member of PACT Ballet tries on her costume and stands patiently as the wardrobe workers adjust the sleeves.

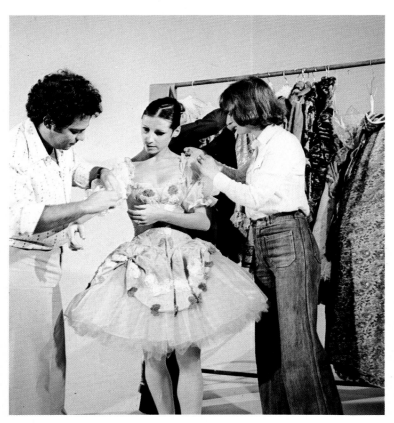

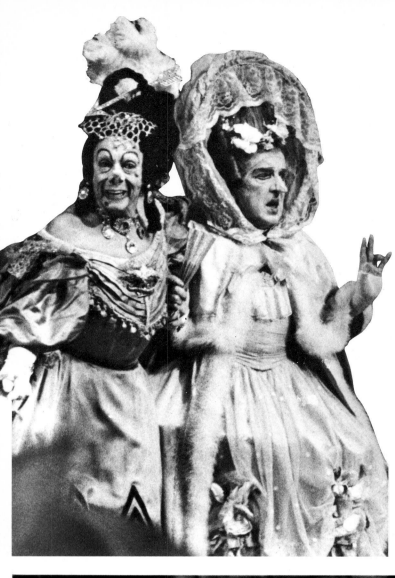

Left: In 1948, Frederick Ashton choreographed his first full-length ballet, Cinderella — a blend of fairy tale and pantomime. The funniest characters are the Ugly Sisters. The two dancers, usually men, who play these parts have to be very good at clowning and comic miming — and they have to wear a lot of make-up. Here, Robert Helpmann as the superior, bossy sister and Ashton himself as the muddly, nervous one.

Below: With greasepaint, Sydney Nolan transforms a dancer into a primitive tribesman for Rite of Spring. The technique of actually painting dancers' bodies is not uncommon, especially in contemporary works.

Bottom: Piglets in a pas de deux from The Tales of Beatrix Potter. Their long snouts made dancing close together rather difficult! Costumes were as authentic as possible. Beatrix Potter wrote during Queen Victoria's reign, so Victorian-style prints and fabrics were chosen for the creatures' clothes while real feathers and fur were used for the tails, heads and bodies. Each squirrel was covered by 50,000 hairs, stuck on in tiny bunches of ten!

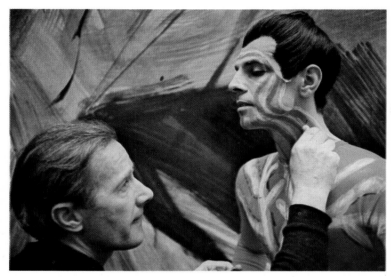

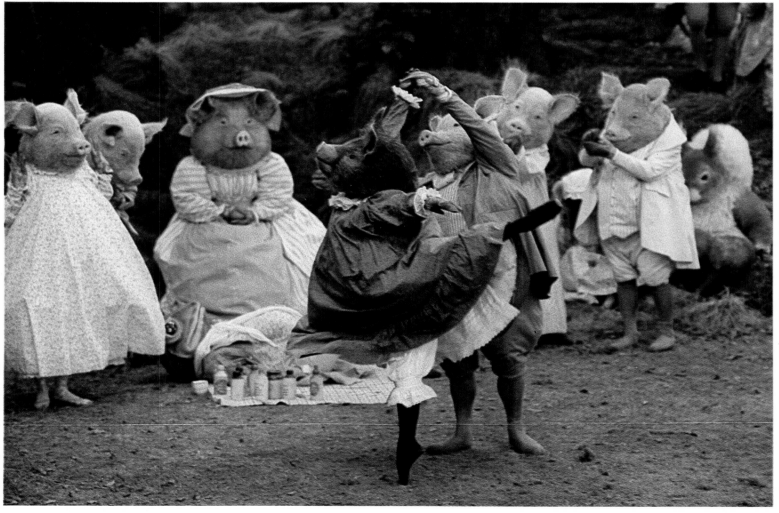

A Ballet Dancer's Life

Dancing is not a nine-to-five job. In fact, it is not much like a job at all: it's more a way of life. A way of life that involves a lot of effort, time, discipline and . . . routine.

The routine begins about ten o'clock in the morning with class. All dancers – even world-famous stars like Anthony Dowell and Natalya Makarova – must practice every day to keep their muscles supple and maintain their technique. Class, lasting two hours, takes place in a studio or rehearsal room. Studios always seem to smell of sweat and rosin – a powder that is rubbed onto the soles of ballet shoes to give a better grip. In class, the dancers – wearing an assortment of clothes: tights, leotards, vests, T-shirts, short tunics, woolly leg-warmers – do *barre* exercises and center work under the direction of the ballet master. Afterwards, a short break: time for a gulp of coffee, a sandwich, or another attempt at a particularly difficult step.

Then back to work: four or five hours of rehearsal. The dancers, still wearing practice clothes and still guided by the ballet master, go through the ballet step by step. Rehearsals usually happen in the studios; often, the soloists work in one studio and the chorus in another. But during the week before a first night the entire cast gets together with the orchestra and rehearses on stage. By the end of the afternoon, around five o'clock, a dancer may have finished for the day – unless he or she is appearing that evening.

The night of a performance

Dancers have to arrive at the theatre well before the start of a performance. They need time to change into their costumes, to put on make-up and to do some exercises to warm the muscles and loosen the joints. (If they went on stage cold and stiff, the results would be disastrous!) Finally, everything is ready. The house lights dim . . . the audience grows quiet . . . the conductor lifts his baton . . . the orchestra starts playing . . . the curtain rises: another performance has begun.

For the dancers, a performance means intense concentration and enormous physical effort; when the curtain falls two hours later, they are very tired. Make-up and costumes come off and then, at last, they can take their aching back, legs and feet home to bed. They have reached the end of an average day: the sort of day that happens all week, except Sundays. Even on tour.

Touring (giving performances in a series of different towns) can be exhausting. To begin with, there is the traveling: long, tedious journeys on Sundays or early weekday mornings. Then, there is the inconvenience of living out of a suitcase. And, there are the working conditions: often, the theatre is small, the dressing rooms are cramped, the stage is slippery . . . No wonder if, behind the scenes, tempers rise.

Why be a dancer?

Why do dancers choose such a hard life? The dancers themselves say they don't choose; rather, they are chosen. Like Rudolf Nureyev. At the age of seven, Rudi went to a ballet for the first time and was immediately bewitched: "From that unforgettable day I was utterly possessed; I had the absolute certitude that I had been born to dance . . . I felt in me the urge, the blind need for dancing and for nothing else."

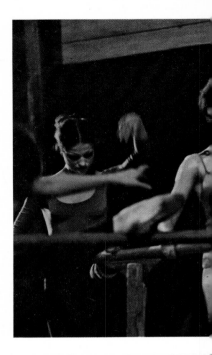

To a dancer, sore feet are a fact of life. Blocked shoes, for *pointe* work, are particularly painful. Dancers try to make wearing them more comfortable by rubbing their feet with rubbing alcohol, sticking first-aid plasters on tender spots, stuffing cotton wool into the toes of the shoes and by putting their heels – with shoes on – under a tap: the shoe shrinks, fits more tightly and so causes less friction. Shoes, normally supplied by the company, are made from satin which is not at all hard-wearing; to make them stronger, the toes are frequently darned before use. Even so, ballet shoes have a very brief existence: a principal (a dancer with a leading role) can easily wear out two pairs of shoes in just one performance, while a chorus member could, with much darning, make a pair last a week. Often, shoes are dyed to match the costume colors.

Maryon Lane, formerly with the Royal Ballet now teaches at the Royal Ballet School.

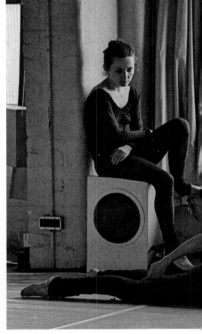

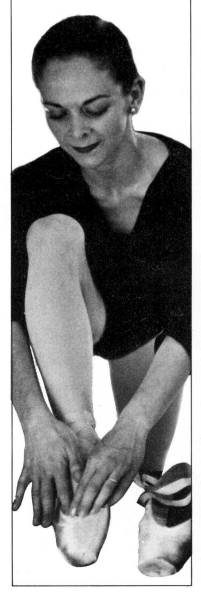

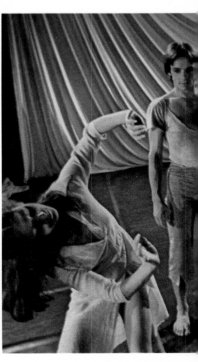

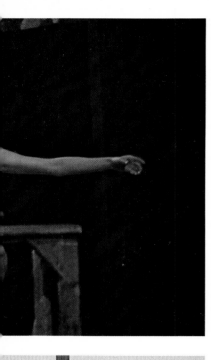

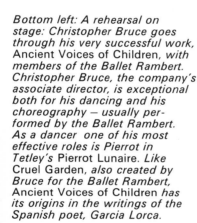

Left: A dancer's day must begin with class. On tour, this can be difficult. Some theatres are so small that there is no room backstage for fifteen or twenty people to do their vital exercises. But somehow, somewhere, class has to happen. A common solution to the space problem is to use the stage itself. The picture shows Ballet Rambert dancers on tour doing classwork on a stage with the help of portable barres.

Center: Long hours of rehearsal are frequently spent waiting. While the choreographer or ballet master practices a solo with one dancer, the others must wait. They do their knitting, read a magazine or massage each other's legs to keep the muscles relaxed and flexible.

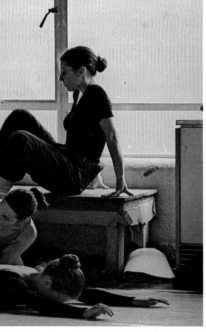

Bottom left: A rehearsal on stage: Christopher Bruce goes through his very successful work, Ancient Voices of Children, *with members of the Ballet Rambert. Christopher Bruce, the company's associate director, is exceptional both for his dancing and his choreography – usually performed by the Ballet Rambert. As a dancer one of his most effective roles is Pierrot in Tetley's* Pierrot Lunaire. *Like* Cruel Garden, *also created by Bruce for the Ballet Rambert,* Ancient Voices of Children *has its origins in the writings of the Spanish poet, Garcia Lorca.*

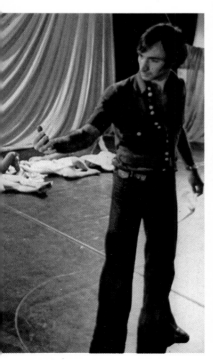

Sadly, a dancing career does not last very long. It begins when the dancer joins a company at seventeen or eighteen and ends before he – or she – is forty. During the early years, dancers usually appear in the *corps de ballet*; it is rare for very young dancers to take the lead. There are, of course, exceptions: by the time she was twenty, Margot Fonteyn had danced Giselle, Odette-Odile (*Swan Lake*) and Aurora (*Sleeping Beauty*). As dancers gain experience, they play more important parts and, in time, may become soloists. A few – those who are outstandingly good – reach the top: they become principals and dance leading roles.

Afterwards what?

Women dancers are generally at their best between thirty and thirty-five; but three or four years later, age catches up with them and they have to retire. Men have to give up even sooner. Again, there are exceptions. Great ballerinas like Galina Ulanova, Alicia Markova and Margot Fonteyn were still dancing in their fifties while some major companies, such as the Bolshoi and the Royal Danish Ballet, have older men for mime and character parts. Most dancers, however, are not so lucky: for them, middle-age means the end of one career and the problem of finding another. Some stay in the dance world as teachers, directors of ballet companies or even as choreographers. Others stay on the stage and take up acting. Others take ordinary, everyday jobs.

The outsider may wonder if being a dancer is worth all the effort: such a long training, such hard work, so many sacrifices for just twenty years' dancing. But dancers know this from the beginning. It does not deter them. They are dedicated. And for dancers, dedication is a must.

Below: Inside the Maryinsky Theatre, Leningrad, home of the world-famous Kirov Ballet. The Maryinsky Theatre was built in 1860, but was not used regularly for ballet performances until 1889. Here, an enthusiastic, excited audience fills the auditorium; in the orchestra pit, the musicians tune their instruments; behind the curtain, the scenery is in position, the lights adjusted, the props assembled; backstage, the dancers, waiting in their costumes, warm up with exercises. At any moment, the lights will go down ready for the magic of another performance.

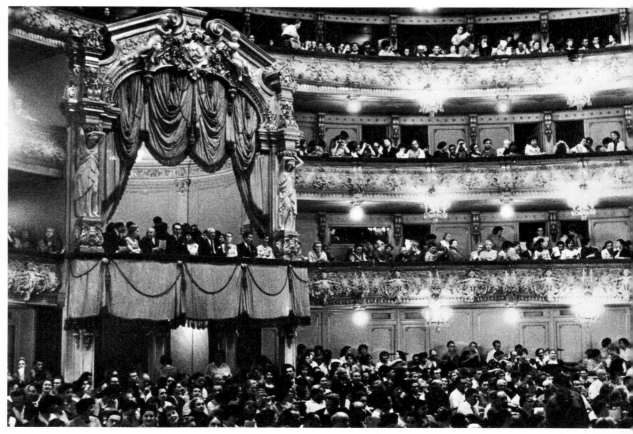

Some Great Companies

Ballet, like music and painting, is not restricted by language: it is truly international. So, not surprisingly, it has spread from its European origins to all parts of the globe and today there are very few countries that do not have at least one ballet company, often more. In spite of their common heritage, the world's ballet companies have developed individual styles of choreography, dancing and décor.

The Royal Danish Ballet

The world's oldest ballet company is the Royal Danish Ballet. It is also one of the most important – thanks to Auguste Bournonville. Bournonville, a friend of Hans Christian Andersen, was director of the company from 1829 to 1877. During that time he had enormous impact: he re-organized the company, trained new dancers, introduced a different teaching method and created over fifty ballets. Among the best are *Napoli*, a folk tale from the Bay of Naples; *Conservatoire*, set in a ballet school; and *Folk Legend*, based on a medieval Danish story. In his ballets, Bournonville always created exciting parts for male dancers – he was himself a brilliant performer – and Danish ballet remains famous for its superb male dancing.

The Royal Danes are proud of the Bournonville heritage and still perform his works. Their repertoire also includes some very modern ballets by Flemming Flindt, an outstanding dancer who became the company's director in 1965. The present director, Henning Kronstam, was previously in charge of the ballet school.

The Bolshoi Ballet

Bolshoi means great: and the Bolshoi Ballet lives up to its name. It is the largest and one of the most important ballet companies in the world. In the days of the Tsar, the Moscow company took second place to the one in St. Petersburg (Leningrad), then the capital. But after the 1917 revolution, when Moscow became the new capital, great efforts were made to turn the Bolshoi into the country's leading company. Top dancers and teachers were transferred from the Kirov (the Leningrad ballet) and many of the finest Kirov productions were re-staged in Moscow, often by their original choreographers. Today the Moscow company is the showcase of Soviet ballet.

The Bolshoi is world-famous for its superb dancing; stars include Maya Plisetskaya, Ekaterina Maximova, Natalia Bessmertnova, Vladimir Vasiliev, Mikhail Lavrovsky and Maris Liepa. Classical ballets such as *Swan Lake*, *Nutcracker* and *Raymonda* form the core of the company's repertoire; among its new works are *Anna Karenina*, *Spartacus* – the story of the slaves' revolt in Ancient Rome, (shown here) and *Ivan the Terrible*, a portrait of the sixteenth-century Tsar who unified Russia.

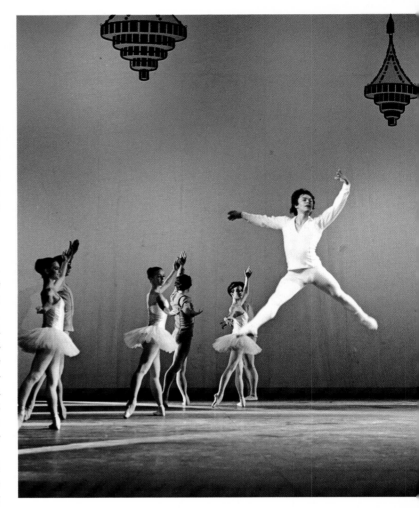

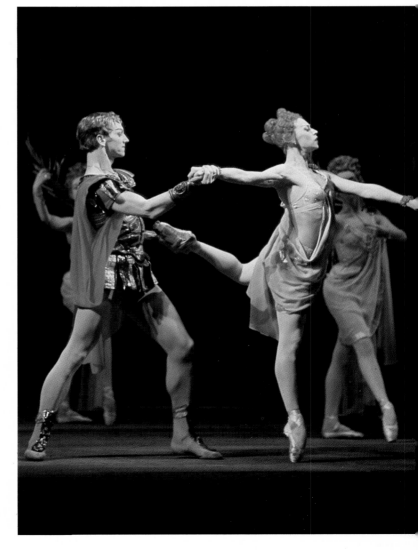

Top: One of the Royal Danes' top dancers, Niels Kehlet, in Études. Études, *an international favorite by the Danish choreographer Harald Lander, imitates a ballet class: it begins with basic steps at the* barre *and ends with some of the most difficult and exciting movements imaginable.*

Right: Maris Liepa, as the tyrant Crassus, with members of the Bolshoi Ballet in Spartacus. *Choreographed by Yuri Grigorovich (the Bolshoi's artistic director and chief choreographer), Spartacus is one of the best-known Soviet ballets. Its music, by the modern composer Aram Khachaturian, is equally popular.*

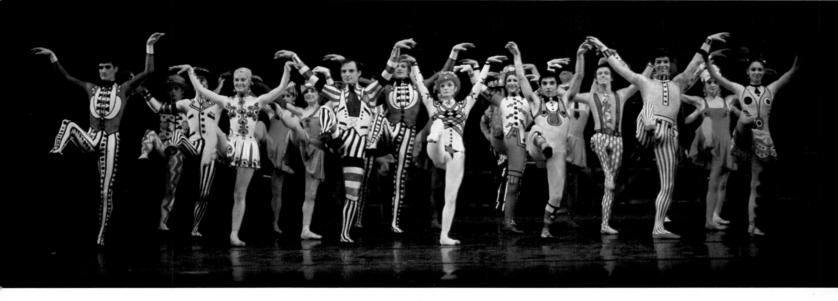

Top: Desmond Kelly and Marion Tait of the Royal Ballet in Elite Syncopations, *a sparkling ragtime romp choreographed by the company's principal choreographer, Kenneth MacMillan. With a ragtime band at the back of the stage, the dancers, dressed in gay carnival costumes, perform a series of brilliant dances, many of them highly amusing. The ballet, first performed in 1974, has become a firm favorite with audiences on both sides of the Atlantic.*

The Royal Ballet

Many years ago in Lima, Peru, a thirteen-year-old English boy saw Pavlova dance. He was thrilled and, from that day, he determined to be a dancer. Frederick Ashton succeeded: he became a dancer and a choreographer. It was mainly as a choreographer that he joined London's new Vic-Wells Ballet in 1935. Working with its founder, Ninette de Valois, he made the Royal Ballet (as it is now called) into one of the world's greatest and best-loved companies. During forty years, Ashton created ballets: masterpieces like *Symphonic Variations, The Dream, La Fille Mal Gardée, Two Pigeons, Enigma Variations* and *A Month in the Country.*

When Ninette de Valois retired as director, Ashton took over, then Kenneth MacMillan. MacMillan, too, is a gifted choreographer and has added important works to the repertoire, including *Anastasia, Elite Syncopations* (shown here), *The Four Seasons* and *Mayerling.* The Royal Ballet has an outstanding repertoire; it also has a tradition of magnificent dancers: Margot Fonteyn, Robert Helpmann, Antoinette Sibley, Lynn Seymour, Merle Park, Anthony Dowell, David Wall . . . The company's stars often appear as guest artists with other groups and, in return, many of the world's top dancers perform at Covent Garden, the Royal Ballet's home.

The Australian Ballet

When Diaghilev died, a new company, based in Monte Carlo, was formed to continue his work. Like the original company, the new *Ballets Russes de Monte Carlo* toured worldwide. At the end of an Australian tour in 1939, one of the dancers, Edouard Borovansky, stayed behind and started his own ballet school and company. For twenty years, the Borovansky Ballet entertained audiences in Australia and New Zealand with a *Ballets Russes*-style repertoire.

After Borovansky's sudden death in 1959, the group disbanded but, two years later, many of its members came together again in the newly-formed Australian Ballet, under the leadership of Peggy van Praagh, a former director of Sadler's Wells. She was later joined by the Australian dancer and choreographer, Robert Helpmann who had been working in Britain.

Together, they built up a repertoire of both classics such as *Swan Lake, Coppélia, Les Sylphides* and *Sleeping Beauty* and new works including *The Display* and *The Merry Widow* (shown here).

Bottom: Members of the Australian Ballet in The Merry Widow, *the first full-length work composed especially for the company. Adapted from the operetta by Franz Lehar, and choreographed by former Royal Ballet principal, Ronald Hynd,* The Merry Widow *was first performed in 1975 and became an immediate success with Australian audiences. This scene occurs in the second act when Hanna (the widow) is giving a party at her villa in Paris. The pavilion in the background is the setting for a rendezvous between two of her guests: Valencienne, the young wife of the Pontevedrian ambassador to France, and Camille, the French attaché. Their secret meeting is interrupted by the unexpected arrival of Valencienne's husband and great confusion follows!*

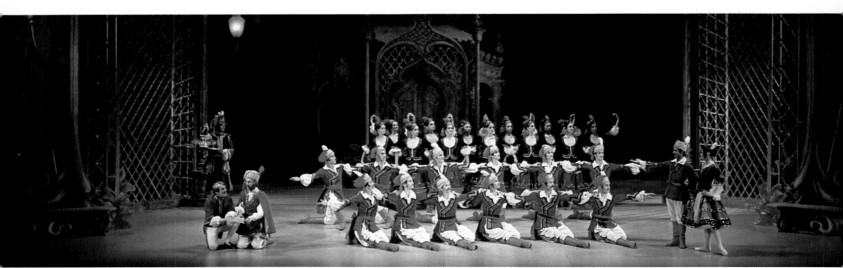

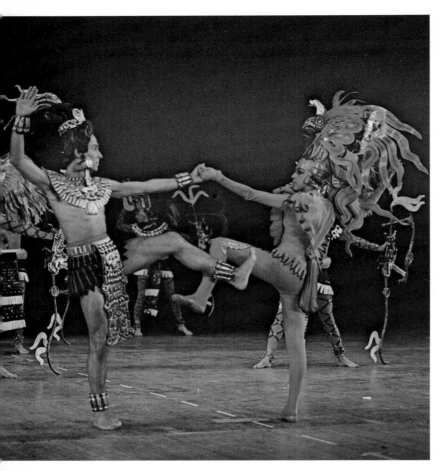

Ballet Folklórico de Mexico

As its name implies, this company has its roots deep in the folk culture of Mexico. Its director and choreographer since its foundation in 1952, Amalia Hernandez, was a ballet teacher with a great interest in the tradional life of her country. She started with a very small company presenting programs on Mexican TV. The company's success led to the government sending it abroad to present Mexican culture to the world. In 1959, it was established as a national group. The ballet now has over 200 dancers, divided between a resident company in Mexico City and groups which tour both within Mexico and abroad.

The Ballet Folklórico has a unique style: combining modern and classical ballet with the rich dance heritage of Mexico. Amalia Hernandez meticulously researches history, art and ceremony before she creates a new ballet, thus making the magnificent scenery and costume as authentic as possible. The company has a repertoire of about twenty of her works as well as classical ballets.

Above: Dancers of the Ballet Folklórico de Mexico in Los Mayas. *Like much of Amalia Hernandez' work, this ballet draws its inspiration from Mexican history and legend: the Mayas were an Indian people who settled in Mexico a thousand years ago.*

Below: Susan Lovell, Homer Bryant and Mel Tomlinson of the Harlem Dance Theatre in Mitchell's Manifestations. *The ballet is based on the biblical story of the Garden of Eden. In preparing for his part as the serpent, Tomlinson bought a real snake so that he could copy its movements.*

Dance Theatre of Harlem

In 1956, when Arthur Mitchell joined the New York City Ballet, he made history: he was the company's first black dancer. In those days, a black dancer in a white chorus was unthinkable, so Mitchell trained as a soloist and became one of the company's star dancers.

Then, in 1968, the black Civil Rights leader Martin Luther King was assassinated. His death affected black people everywhere. Mitchell was no exception. Inspired by the ideals of the Civil Rights movement – equality for blacks – he devoted himself to bringing ballet to his own race. He went to Harlem and started a school of classical dance. Two years later, he founded the world's only black classical ballet company: the Dance Theatre of Harlem.

Although it is still a very young dance group, the Dance Theatre of Harlem is amazingly successful. Its repertoire is a mix of classical and ethnic dance and includes works by Balanchine — Ballet Master of the New York City Ballet, by Mitchell himself and by William Scott, a member of the company.

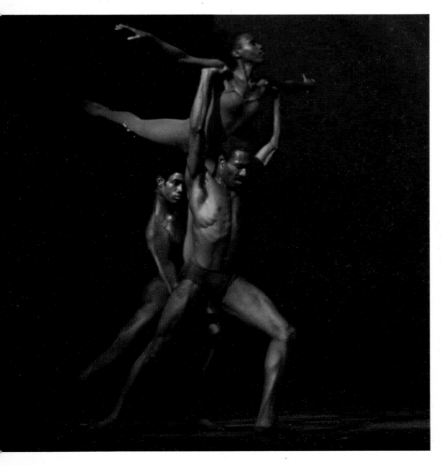

The Stuttgart Ballet

West Germany is one of the few countries without a national ballet company. And although there are over sixty ballet groups attached to opera houses in the main towns, most are small and not very important. Both the Hamburg State Opera Ballet and the Berlin Opera Ballet are known internationally. The Tanz-Forum of Cologne has a world-wide reputation for its modern repertoire. But the outstanding company is the Stuttgart Ballet.

Before 1960, the Stuttgart company resembled other provincial companies. Then John Cranko arrived and, within a few years, the Stuttgart ballet became world-famous. Cranko, a South African, was an exceptional choreographer. He created his first ballet in Cape Town, then moved to London to work for Sadler's Wells: two of his biggest hits were *Pineapple Poll* and *Prince of the Pagodas*. At Stuttgart he brought in top dancers, among them the exquisite Brazilian ballerina, Marcia Haydée; he founded a ballet school – now one of the best in Europe; and he built up an impressive repertoire.

In 1973, Cranko died suddenly, but the Stuttgart Ballet continues its remarkable and dynamic career under the guidance of Marcia Haydée.

The New York City Ballet

In 1933, Lincoln Kirstein — author, editor, and patron of the arts — met Russian dancer-choreographer George Balanchine for the first time in a London kitchen. Out of that meeting was born one of the great ballet companies of the world — the New York City Ballet.

In New York the two founded the School of American Ballet and a touring troupe, American Ballet. The troupe became Ballet Caravan in 1936 and Ballet Society in 1946. Through Kirstein's general management and the artistic direction of Balanchine and Jerome Robbins, audiences were treated to a refreshing, and distinctively American, classical ballet. In 1948 the New York City Ballet gave its first performance at City Center. In 1964 it found a permanent home in Lincoln Center.

The company's fast-paced, dynamic repertoire reflects the taste and style of its main choreographer. Balanchine ballets are built on music as their titles often show — *Allegro Brillante, Opus 34, Symphony in C.* Steps, however, are not merely danced to the music; they seem to grow out of it. Many pieces are plotless, focusing on movement rather than story. In fact, despite its basis in classical dance, the company often startles audiences with unusual, and even unconventional, ballets.

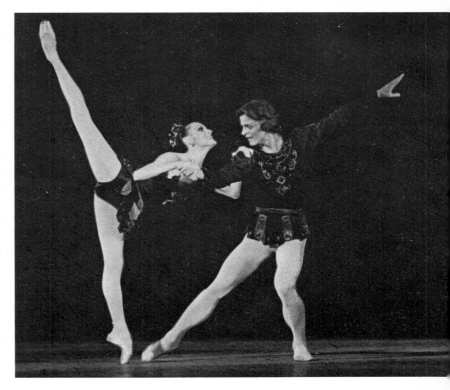

Above: Patricia McBride and Mikhail Baryshnikov of the New York City Ballet in Rubies, *part of Balanchine's plotless ballet,* Jewels.

Ballet Théâtre Contemporain

In 1968 the French Ministry of Culture founded the Ballet Théâtre Contemporain. The young company was charged with presenting new ballets which reflect contemporary thought and bring together musicians, designers, dancers and even sculptors in a communal effort.

The company started its life in Amiens, but four years later moved to Angers. From there it tours the whole of France and travels to many other countries.

Its ballets (under the direction of Jean-Albert Cartier and the choreographer Françoise Adret) are up-to-the-minute creations, representing new trends in thought and in social life.

The Ballet Théâtre Contemporain soon made its mark with its vivid and imaginative programs and varied repertoire. The company's work is constantly changing as it strives to reflect the changing world to its audiences.

The company is very concerned with "taking dance to the people", and uses all sorts of methods – discussions, lectures, film shows – to reach the widest possible audience.

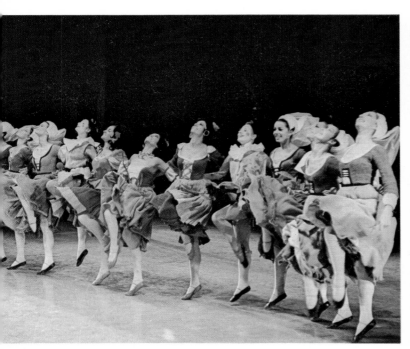

During his twelve years as director of the Stuttgart company, Cranko added fifty new ballets to its repertoire, including Romeo and Juliet, *set to Prokofiev's music (above),* Onegin *and* The Taming of the Shrew.

Right: Members of the Ballet Théâtre Contemporain in Hopop, *a lively creation by Dirk Sanders, a Dutch dancer and choreographer who has composed several works for the company.*

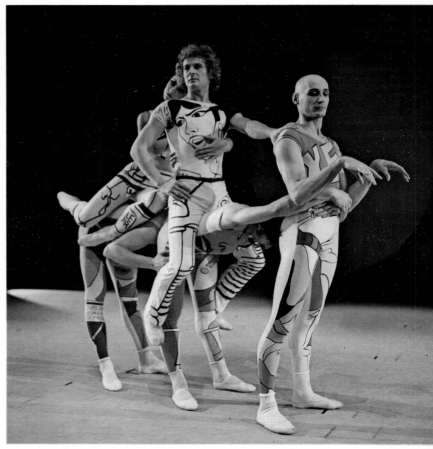

Some Great Ballets

Ballet is very up to date: each year, hundreds of new ballets are created and every company's repertoire includes contemporary works. But not all today's ballets will be seen by tomorrow's audiences, just as many of yesterday's productions are now unknown. Only good ballets survive: the ones that audiences enjoy watching and dancers like performing. Bad ballets are seldom staged and soon forgotten. A few well-known ballets are presented here. Some have already passed the test of time, others – more modern – are expected to pass it when their turn comes.

The Nutcracker

Danced to Tchaikovsky's sparkling music, *The Nutcracker* (1892), is performed more often than any other ballet. The curtain rises on a Christmas party at the home of Clara and Fritz. When all the guests have arrived, presents are handed out to the excited children. Clara is particularly delighted with one gift: a Nutcracker, shaped like a soldier. At the end of the party, Clara and Fritz are put to bed and are soon fast asleep. Later that night, however, the little girl wakes up and creeps downstairs to the darkened drawing-room to play with her Nutcracker. But strange things happen in the drawing-room: the Nutcracker grows bigger, then comes alive and so does a regiment of toy soldiers. Just in time! For, to Clara's horror, an army of mice led by the ferocious Mouse King appears. The brave Nutcracker leaps to Clara's defense. He summons the toy soldiers and a fierce battle rages. The Nutcracker and the Mouse King fight a duel. Sadly, the courageous Nutcracker seems to be losing when Clara suddenly acts: she snatches off her slipper and throws it at the evil King; for a second, the Mouse is distracted and the Nutcracker is able to kill him. In this moment of victory, the Nutcracker is transformed into a handsome prince and takes Clara on a magic journey through the Land of Snow to the Kingdom of Sweets. The Sugar Plum Fairy welcomes them and announces that a great festival of dance is to be held in Clara's honor. Then follows a wonderful entertainment: dancers from all parts of the world – Spain, Arabia, Turkey, China, Russia – perform for Clara and her Nutcracker prince; the festivities finish with a grand *pas de deux* and a final waltz. As the dancing ends, Clara feels terribly sleepy . . . When she wakes up, she is alone at home with her Nutcracker doll. Was it all a dream?

Top: The London Festival Ballet's production of The Nutcracker. *This popular work, performed by the Festival Ballet in its early days, is still regularly staged by the company at Christmas. The Festival Ballet, founded by Alicia Markova and Anton Dolin in 1950, is world-famous — especially for its superb presentations of many full-length classical works. The present director is Beryl Grey, formerly one of Britain's outstanding ballerinas.*

Right: Margarethe Schanne as the forest sprite and Henning Kronstam as James in the Royal Danish Ballet's production of La Sylphide. *Although the original ballet was created by Taglioni for his daughter, Marie, the version of* La Sylphide *which is seen today was choreographed in 1836 by Auguste Bournonville. Bournonville, director of the Danish company for fifty years, was one of the most influential and talented figures in the history of ballet.*

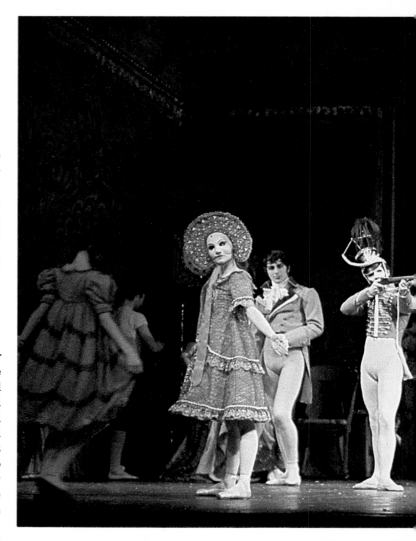

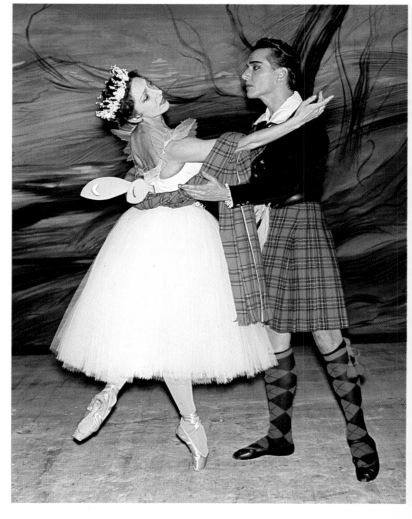

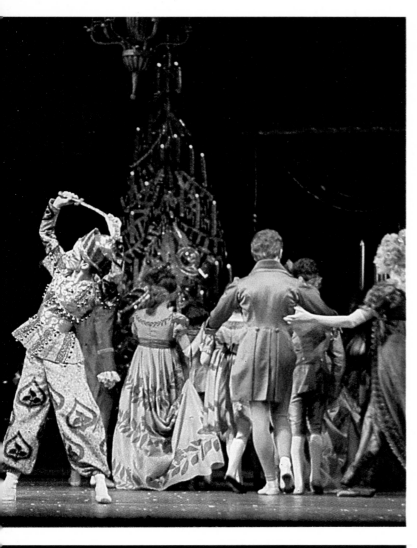

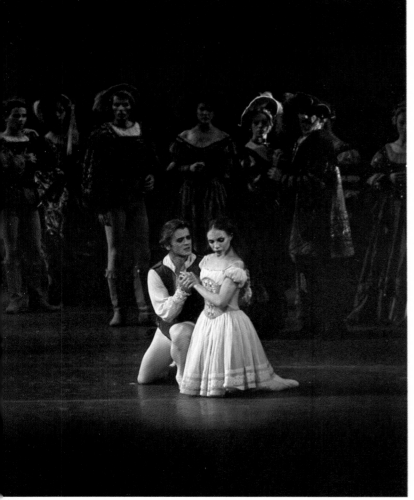

La Sylphide

Created for Marie Taglioni by her father, the original *La Sylphide* (1832), was the first great romantic ballet.

The story takes place in a Scottish village where James, a young farmer, is about to marry a local girl, Effie. The day before the wedding, a beautiful forest sprite – the sylphide – appears in James' house and the young man immediately falls in love with her. James is now torn between Effie and the sylphide, who contines to haunt him. While the young couple prepare for the wedding – with the sprite flitting in and out – an old woman arrives. This is Madge, a witch, who tells Effie that she will never marry James. Madge's words anger James and he drives her out of the house. The sprite, however, eventually succeeds in luring James away into the forest.

In the forest, James is blissfully happy: the sprite brings him gifts and they dance together. But disaster is near: Madge, determined to get her revenge, is plotting against James. With her sister witches Madge makes a poisoned shawl which she gives to James. He, in turn, hands the shawl to the sprite who eagerly puts it on. The evil spell begins to work: her wings drop off and she dies in James' arms.

At this moment a wedding procession passes in the distance: Effie, thinking James gone for ever, has married his rival, Gurn. Seeing this, James collapses with grief: he has lost both his loves.

Giselle

A French poet fell in love with an Italian ballerina and for her he wrote one of the greatest-ever ballet stories. The poet was Théophile Gautier; the ballerina, Carlotta Grisi; the ballet, *Giselle* (1841).

The story opens in a Rhineland village on the edge of a forest. Giselle, the prettiest girl in the village, falls madly in love with Loys, a peasant boy who has just arrived in the area. Giselle sees more and more of Loys and has no time for Hilarion, a young woodman who wants to marry her. Hilarion is suspicious of the stranger and one day he breaks into Loys' cottage where he discovers a nobleman's sword: Loys is really the Duke Albrecht. Meanwhile, a hunting party has stopped in the village for refreshment. The party includes Princess Bathilde, Albrecht's fiancée, and when Hilarion reveals Loys' true identity, Bathilde confirms it. Giselle is so shocked by the news that she goes mad with grief and dies.

The scene changes to the forest glade where Giselle is buried. At night the forest is haunted by Wilis, the spirits of young girls betrayed in love. Any man who sees them is forced to dance until he is exhausted and dies. When Hilarion visits Giselle's grave, he is surrounded by the ghostly spirits and dances to his death. Then Albrecht comes. Giselle herself is now a Wili, and Myrtha, the cruel Wili Queen, orders her to make the duke dance until he, too, dies. But Giselle still loves Albrecht. She keeps him dancing until dawn, when the Wilis' power comes to an end. As day filters through the trees, the Wilis return to their graves leaving Albrecht alone, but alive – saved through Giselle's deep love.

Left: Mikhail Baryshnikov (Albrecht) and Gelsey Kirkland (Giselle) with members of the American Ballet Theatre in Giselle.
Mikhail Baryshnikov was born in 1948 in the USSR, trained in Leningrad, and became one of the Kirov's most brilliant artists. In 1974, while on tour in Canada, he decided to stay in the West. He has since appeared with many companies, especially the American Ballet Theatre and more recently Balanchine's New York City Ballet. He is acclaimed world-wide as the greatest dancer of his generation. His skill is astonishing: when he leaps he seems to hang in the air. He brings an exciting sense of theatre to all his roles.

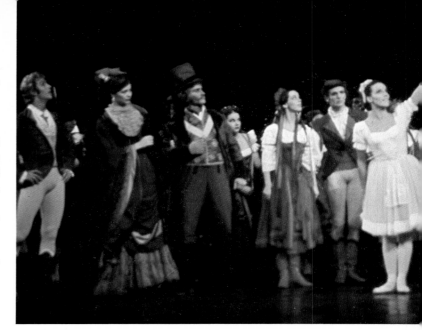

Coppélia

With enchanting music especially composed by Delibes, *Coppélia* (1870) has a happy story.

The action centers round a village girl, Swanilda, her boyfriend, Franz, an old toymaker, Dr. Coppélius, and the beautiful Coppélia who sometimes appears at the toymaker's window. Franz is very attracted to Coppélia and, whenever he sees her, he bows and blows her kisses. Franz' flirting annoys Swanilda and makes her jealous of the mysterious Coppélia. One day, as Dr. Coppélius is crossing the village square, he drops his key. Swanilda and her friends find it and decide to explore the old man's house.

Inside the house, Swanilda and friends find many strange silent figures. At first, the girls are frightened, then they realize the figures are only dolls. They laugh when they open a cupboard and discover Coppélia – just another doll. Their fun is stopped by an angry Dr. Coppélius; he chases them out, but Swanilda hides in the cupboard and puts on Coppélia's clothes.

No sooner has Dr. Coppélius sat down than Franz comes in, looking for the lovely Coppélia. At first the toymaker is cross, then he has an idea: he has always wanted to make one of his dolls come to life by giving it a human spirit and he now decides to experiment. He drugs Franz, brings out Coppélia (really Swanilda) then casts his spells. To the old man's great joy, the magic works: the doll gradually comes alive and starts to dance.

But the toymaker's delight soon turns to horror: Swanilda tears up his book of spells, knocks over the other dolls, wakes Franz from his drugged sleep and finally flings open the cupboard to reveal the lifeless Coppélia.

The story ends with a village festival at which engaged couples, including Swanilda and Franz, receive purses full of gold coins.

La Fille Mal Gardée

La Fille Mal Gardée (1960) is a modern version, by Ashton, of an old ballet. Set in France, the story is about Lise, the daughter of Widow Simone, and her love for Colas, a young farmer. Unfortunately, Simone wants Lise to marry Alain, the idiot son of Thomas, a rich vineyard-owner.

It is dawn and Simone's farm is coming to life: the laborers leave for the harvest fields while Lise begins her day's work. Colas joins her but the lovers are interrupted by Simone who chases him away. The couple outwit Simone and contrive another brief meeting. Later Thomas calls with Alain to discuss the marriage.

In the fields, the farmworkers and Colas are celebrating the end of the harvest. Simone, Thomas, Lise and Alain join the festivities. While everyone is merrymaking, the lovers escape together, but, inevitably, are hauled back by Simone.

Back home, Simone dozes off and Lise talks with Colas through the locked door. The harvesters bring in sheaves of corn, and Simone goes out to get them a celebration drink. Immediately, Colas appears from under the sheaves. Once again the two young people declare their love; once again they are interrupted by Simone. As soon as Lise hears Simone, she tells Colas to hide in her bedroom. Simone, ever suspicious, locks Lise in the same room until Thomas and Alain come to sign the wedding contract. The two men arrive, the contract is signed and Alain is sent to Lise's room to claim his bride. There he finds Lise and Colas in each other's arms. Thomas, furious, tears up the contract and storms out dragging Alain with him. The lovers plead with Simone; eventually she relents and agrees to their marriage.

This ballet is sometimes known as *Vain Precautions* or, a closer translation, *The Unchaperoned Daughter*.

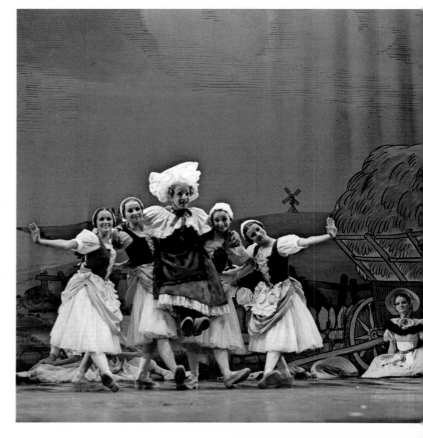

Above: Ronald Emblen as Widow Simone in La Fille Mal Gardée, *performed by the Sadler's Wells Royal Ballet. In the fields, the workers have finished the harvest and here Simone is doing her lively clog dance as part of the general merrymaking.*

Right: Petrushka, danced by members of the Royal Ballet with Rudolf Nureyev (right) in the title role. Nureyev began his dancing career in Leningrad and during only three years with the Kirov he established himself as a phenomenal artist. But in 1961, during a European tour, he decided to leave the USSR. Since then, as guest star with many companies, he has dazzled audiences all over the world. In this production of Petrushka, *the ballerina's part is taken by the South African, Nadia Nerina.*

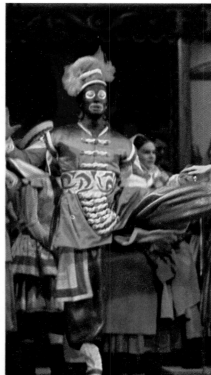

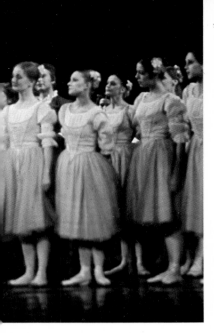

Left: Carole Hill with dancers of the London Festival Ballet in Coppélia. *Thanks to its delightful story and sparkling music,* Coppélia *is a traditional favorite with the public and as such is frequently performed by companies everywhere.*

Below: A production of Pineapple Poll *by the Royal Ballet. This scene occurs when Captain Belaye's gunboat,* Hot Cross Bun, *is back in port after the voyage; the real crew go on board and angrily discover the true identity of the so-called sailors.*

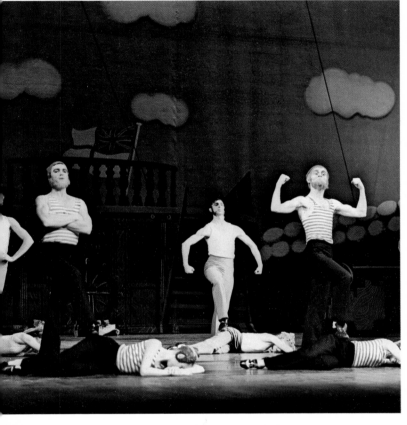

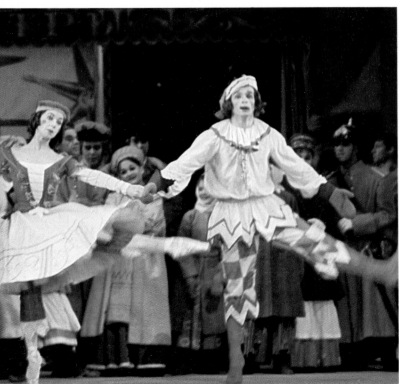

Pineapple Poll

Danced to Arthur Sullivan's music *Pineapple Poll* (1951) is a lively, light-hearted story set in Portsmouth, England.

One afternoon some sailors gather with their girlfriends in front of a quayside inn. They are joined by Poll, a pretty trinket-seller. As she moves from group to group, she is watched by the adoring Jasper. The heartless girl just mocks him. Then Captain Belaye, commander of the gunboat *Hot Cross Bun*, arrives. He is so handsome that all the girls instantly fall in love with him. Belaye ignores them. He has come to meet his fiancée, Blanche, and her chattering aunt, Mrs. Dimple.

That evening Poll, dreaming only of Belaye, goes down to the quay and gazes sadly at his ship, which must soon leave port. The sight of a sailor's uniform lying on the ground gives her an idea. She puts it on and goes on board. She will sail with Belaye disguised as a member of his crew. Jasper comes looking for Poll. To his horror he finds her clothes in a heap on the quayside and imagines she has drowned herself for love of Belaye.

During the voyage, Belaye finds his crew a little strange, especially Poll who faints at the sound of a cannon. Once the *Hot Cross Bun* gets back to Portsmouth, however, the captain forgets his odd crew and rushes ashore. His return, with Blanche, in her wedding dress, and Aunt Dimple, almost causes a riot. Poll tears off her uniform and declares her love for him. To everyone's amazement, the rest of the crew follow her example. They are all girls in disguise.

Then the real crew, led by Jasper, arrives. The sailors are angry with their sweethearts for running off to sea, but are persuaded to forgive and forget.

All ends happily: Belaye is made an admiral, Jasper becomes the new captain of *Hot Cross Bun* and Poll decides to marry him after all.

Petrushka

Diaghilev's masterpiece was *Petrushka* (1911). The ballet in four scenes was choreographed by Michel Fokine to Stravinsky's music. The original décor was by Benois.

It is set at the Butterweek Fair, held each Lent in St. Petersburg. In a crowded square is a puppet booth. The show is about to begin; people eagerly gather round. The curtains open and there are three puppets: the pretty Ballerina, the sad, shabby Petrushka and the magnificent Moor. But these are no ordinary puppets: as the Showman waves his wand the wooden figures come to life.

After the performance, the Showman shuts the puppets away in separate compartments. But he cannot undo his magic: the wooden dolls still behave like humans. Petrushka is very miserable. He is desperately in love with the Ballerina, but he is too ugly and awkward to please her. As he lies unhappily on the floor, the door opens. The Ballerina comes in. Petrushka, overjoyed, declares his love. The heartless Ballerina just laughs. He tries to impress her by performing marvelous jumps and turns; she pretends to be frightened and runs away. She then visits the Moor, who is lolling on a heap of splendid silk cushions, and flirts with him. The Moor is delighted and has just embraced her when Petrushka rushes in. He hurls himself at the Moor and they fight fiercely. The thin little Petrushka is no match for the bully who chases him out into the square. There, the Moor raises his scimitar and, with one savage blow, kills Petrushka. The horrified crowd is calmed by the Showman who explains that the victim really is only a puppet for sawdust, not blood, pours from the wound. The Showman drags the broken puppet towards the booth. Suddenly, he hears a fearful shriek and, looking up, sees the ghost of Petrushka cursing him from the top of the booth.

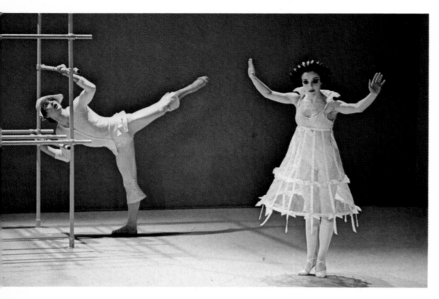

Pierrot Lunaire

Glen Tetley's first ballet, *Pierrot Lunaire* (1962), uses traditional figures that trace their origin back to the theatre of ancient Rome.

The three characters are: the white clown of innocence (Pierrot), the dark clown of experience (Brighella) and deceitful woman (Columbine). The ballet opens with Pierrot, all in white, lazily swinging on a tower of white scaffolding. His dreams fade away with the arrival of Columbine who treats him pleasantly. Pierrot is overjoyed but, as he tries to kiss her, she slaps him and runs away. When she returns, full of scorn, the dejected Pierrot grovels on the ground. Then Brighella, in dark clothes, arrives and starts to play with Pierrot. But there is not much fun in the game as Brighella is a tough, conceited bully. Next Brighella and Columbine turn on Pierrot: they tease and taunt him, attach cords to make him their puppet and pull off his white clothes. Defeated, Pierrot lies miserably in a heap. The other two dance around jubilantly, then leap triumphantly up his tower. Pierrot struggles to his feet, staggers to the scaffolding and slowly climbs up; there, he embraces Columbine and Brighella in forgiveness.

Tetley's ballet shows how Pierrot, the innocent dreamer, is hurt by experience at the cruel hands of Columbine and Brighella but finds the strength to forgive them and to accept the challenge of life. The theme is like *Petrushka*, except that Petrushka conquers only in death while Pierrot triumphs in life.

Swan Lake

The greatest of the Tchaikovsky ballets is *Swan Lake* (1895).

The ballet opens with Prince Siegfried's twenty-first birthday: now he has come of age he knows he must marry and must choose a bride at tomorrow's Grand Ball. This thought depresses the prince and, as dusk falls, he decides to distract himself by going hunting. Beside the lake he watches a flight of swans dropping down to the water. As the birds glide towards him, Siegfried is amazed to see the leading swan change into a beautiful woman. She tells him that she is Odette, queen of a group of maidens who have been bewitched by the magician, von Rothbart. Under his evil spell they are condemned to live as swans by day but become human again at night. Siegfried falls deeply in love with Odette and learns the spell can only be broken if he promises to love her and no-one else. Together, they dance tenderly until dawn steals over the lake; then Odette, once more a swan, glides away.

At the Grand Ball, Siegfried hardly notices the young girls presented to him: all his thoughts are with Odette. Suddenly, two unexpected guests are announced: von Rothbart, disguised as a nobleman, and his daughter Odile. By her father's magic, Odile appears to be Odette and succeeds in captivating Siegfried. The prince asks her to marry him and swears his eternal love. Immediately, von Rothbart and Odile reveal their true identity and, with mocking laughter, disappear in a cloud of smoke. Siegfried, distraught at having broken his promise to Odette, rushes to the lakeside to find the Swan Queen. There, he begs her forgiveness and they are joyfully reunited. But their happiness is soon threatened: von Rothbart appears and says that Siegfried must keep his oath and marry Odile. To escape the magician's power, the two lovers plunge to their death in the lake. Their sacrifice breaks the spell: von Rothbart dies, the swan-maidens become human again and Siegfried and Odette are united for evermore in a paradise beneath the waters of the lake.

Top: Rudolf Nureyev as Pierrot and Lucy Burge, of the Ballet Rambert, as Columbine in Pierrot Lunaire. *Although the ballet has only three characters, it provides a very moving – and honest – picture of human nature.*

Below: The London Festival Ballet in Swan Lake *with Liliana Belfiore as Odette and Nicholas Johnson as Siegfried. The lyrical, sensitive movements of the* corps de ballet *form an exceptionally beautiful background to the soloists.*

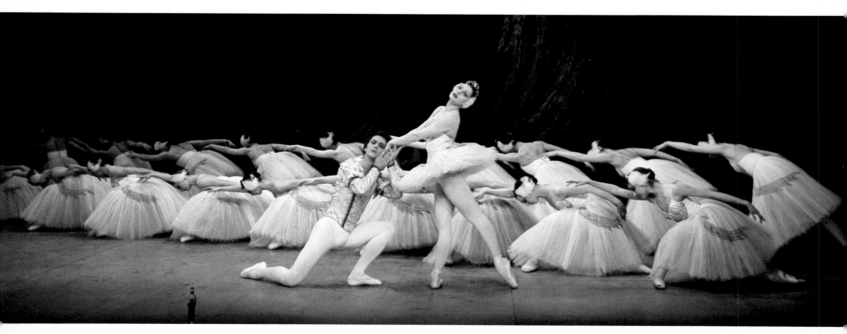

Index

ACKNOWLEDGEMENTS

Design and illustrations:
Dave Nash.

Cover design: Kay Eglise.

Picture research: Penny J. Warn.

Cover, endpapers and title page:
Jesse Davis

Illustrations in text:
Australian Ballet Company:
page 6 top, page 37 bottom.
BBC: page 35 bottom left.
Institute of Choreology: page
28 bottom right. Benesh
Movement Notation
copyright 1955 Rudolf
Benesh.
Anthony Crickmay: pages 9
and 13.
Jesse Davis: 12 center, 16,
17, 25 bottom right,
26 bottom, 27, 28 top and
bottom, 32 top, 36 top, 38
top and bottom, 39 bottom
left and right, 40 bottom, 41
bottom, 42 top, center left
and right.
Zoë Dominic: 6 top, 15
bottom right, 20, 23, 24
bottom, 25 bottom left, 26
top, 29 top and bottom
right, 30 top, 33 top and
center, 34, 35 bottom right,
37 top, 40 top, 42 bottom,
44.
Danish Tourist Board: page 8.
E.M.I.: 6 center, 30 bottom,
33 bottom.
Giraudon: page 10.
Malcolm Hoare: Contents
page, bottom left, 15
bottom left, 25 top, 29
bottom left, 35 top and
center.
Mander and Mitchenson:
page 12 bottom.
Monarch Films: page 15 top.
Novosti: 12 top left, 18, 36
bottom.
National Ballet of Canada:
page 31 bottom.
PACT Ballet Company,
South Africa: 24 center, 26
left, 32 bottom.
Sadler's Wells Theatre: 7, 25
center, 31 top.
Victoria and Albert Museum:
page 11.
Zefa (UK) Ltd: page 14.

Editor: Deborah Manley.

Advisor: Tony Barlow,
London Festival Ballet

A
Agon 32
American Ballet Theatre 41
Anastasia 14, 37
Anatomy Lesson 27
Ancient Voices of Children 35
Anna Karenina 36
Arabesques 22
Ashton, Sir Frederick 7, 17, 25,
    26, 29, 30, 33, 37, 42
Assemblés 23
Attitudes 22
Australian Ballet 7, 37

B
Balanchine, George 13, 14, 26, 27
    28, 29, 38
Ballet as a career 34–35
Ballet Comique de la Reine 10
Ballet de la Nuit 10
Ballet Folklórico de Mexico 38
Ballet Rambert 6, 25, 29, 35, 44
Ballet school 15–18
Ballet du XXe Siécle 14
Ballet Théâtre Contemporain 39
Ballets Russes 9, 13, 14, 18, 32, 37
Barre 10, 18, 20, 21, 22, 25, 35, 36
Baryshnikov, Mikhail 16, 41
Battements 20, 21
Beauchamp, Pierre 10, 19
Béjart, Maurice 14
Benesh, Rudolf 28
Benois, Alexandre 32, 43
Bolshoi Ballet 18, 35, 36
Borovansky, Eduoard 37
Bournonville, Auguste 9, 36, 40
Boutique Fantasque 13
Brandenburg 2 and 4 28
Bruce, Christopher 35
Burne, Gary 26
Bush Davies School 16

C
Camargo, Marie 11
Card Game 26
Cartier, Jean-Albert 39
Center practice 22
Changements 23
Checkmate 27
Chopiniana 18
Choreographer and choreography
    27–29 and passim
Cinderella 33
Conservatoire 36
Coppélia 14, 24, 30, 42
Corps de ballet 11, 35, 44
Costumes 14, 25, 30, 33
Covent Garden 17, 37
Cranko, John 27, 28, 38, 39
Cruel Garden 14, 35
Cunningham, Merce 13

D
Dance Theatre of Harlem 27, 38
Dances at a Gathering 15, 30
Degas, Edgar 10
Delicate Balance 31
Developpés 21
Diaghilev, Serge 9, 11, 13, 32, 37
    43
Display, The 37
Dolin, Anton 9, 13, 40
Don Quixote 27
Double work 24
Dowell, Anthony 20, 34, 37
Dream, The 14, 37
Duncan, Isadora 13
Dutch National Ballet 39
Dying Swan 12

E
Echappés 22
Elite Syncopations 6, 27, 37
Embrace Tiger and Return to
    Mountain 27
Enigma Variations 28, 30, 37
Etudes 4, 36

F
Falla, Manuel de 13
Fancy Free 15
Fille Mal Gardée 31, 37, 42
Firebird 13
Flindt, Flemming 8, 9, 36
Floor work 25
Fokine, Michel 9, 12, 13, 18, 43
Folk Legend 36
Fonteyn, Margot 16, 26, 35, 37
Fouettés 22
Four Seasons 37

G
Giselle 13, 14, 23, 32, 35, 41
Goldberg Variations 15
Graham, Martha 12, 13, 16, 25
Grant, Alexander 31
Grey, Beryl 9, 40
Grigorovich, Yuri 36

H
Harlem Dance Theatre 27, 38
Haydée, Marcia 28, 38
Helpmann, Robert 33, 37
Hernandez, Amalia 38
Hopop 39
Hynd, Ronald 37

I, J, K
Imperial Ballet 11, 13, 16, 18
Ivan the Terrible 14, 36
Jetés 23
Jewels 32
Karsavina, Tamara 12, 13
Kehlet, Niels 36
Khatchaturian, Aram 36
Kirov Ballet 16, 18, 35, 36, 41
Kronstam, Henning 36, 40

L
Laban, Rudolf von 28
Labnotation 28
Lament of the Waves 29
Lander, Harald 36
L'apres midi d'un Faune 13
Lehar, Franz 37
Liebeslieder Waltzes 14
Liepa, Maris 36
Lifar, Serge 13, 32
London Contemporary Dance Theatre 9
London Festival Ballet 9, 13, 23,
    24, 32, 35, 40, 43, 44
Los Mayas 38

M
MacMillan, Kenneth 28, 30, 37
Manifestations 38
Margerite and Armand 26
Markarova, Natalya 16, 34
Markova, Alicia 9, 13, 15, 35, 40
Maryinsky Theatre 35
Massine, Leonid 13
Mayerling 37
Merry Widow 37
Mitchell, Arthur 38
Modern dance 25
Monotones II 25
Month in the Country 37
Music and ballet 28–29 and passim

N
Napoli 13, 16, 36
National Ballet of Canada 31
National dance 15,17
Netherlands Dans Theater 39
New York City Ballet 13, 15, 29
    38
Nijinsky, Vaslav 12, 13, 14
Nikolais, Alwin 25
Nikolais Dance Theatre 25
Noah's Minstrels 7
Noir et blanc 32
Nongause 26
Notation 28
Noverre, Jean-Georges 11
Nureyev, Rudolf 16, 26, 34, 42, 44
Nutcracker 11, 14, 17, 27, 28, 30,
    32, 36, 40

O
Ondine 26
Onegin 39

P
PACT Ballet 24, 26, 32
Paris Opera Ballet 10, 13
Pas de deux 11, 16, 24, 27, 33
Patineurs, Les 17
Paul Taylor Dance Company 7
Pavlova, Anna 12, 13, 37
Perm choreographic school 18
Peter and the Wolf 28
Petipa, Marius 11, 27
Petrushka 32, 43, 44
Phaedra 12
Pierrot Lunaire 30, 44
Pineapple Poll 14, 32, 38, 43
Pirouettes 22
Pliés 20
Point work 24
Positions, of arms 19
    of feet 19
Posture 19
Praagh, Peggy van 37
Prince of the Pagodas 38
Prodigal Son 13, 27
Properties 31

R
Rambert, Marie 13, 14
Raymonda 36
Revelations 27
Rite of Spring 14, 28, 30, 33
Robbins, Jerome 15, 30
Romantic movement, The 11
Romeo and Juliet 39
Rond de jambe 21
Royal Ballet 6, 13, 14, 17, 20, 25,
    28, 29, 30, 31, 34, 37, 42, 43
Royal Danish Ballet 8, 9, 16, 35,
    36

S
Sacre du Printemps, see Rite
    of Spring
Sadler's Wells 9, 13, 31, 38
Sanders, Dirk 39
Scapino Ballet 39
Scenery 14, 25, 30–31
Serenade 14, 28
Shoes, ballet 17, 34
Sleeping Beauty 11, 12, 24, 27,
    28, 35, 37
Song of the Earth 28
Soubresauts 23
Spartacus 32, 36
Spectre de la Rose 12
Stars and Stripes 14
Stretching 21
Stuttgart Ballet 15, 26, 27, 38
Swan Lake 11, 17, 22, 27, 30,
    35, 36, 44
Sylphide, La 11, 30, 32, 40, 41
Sylphides, Les 9, 13, 18, 32, 37
Symphonic Variations 30, 37

T
Taglioni, Marie 10, 11, 41
Tales of Beatrix Potter 7, 14, 30, 33
Taming of the Shrew 14, 30, 39
Taylor, Paul 7, 13
Tchaikovsky, Pyotr 11, 14, 28, 30,
    40, 44
Tensile Involvement 25
Tetley, Glen 13, 30, 39, 44
Three Cornered Hat 13, 17, 32
Toronto Dance Theatre 25, 31
Triumph of Death 9
Turn-out 19
Two Pigeons 27, 30, 37

U, V, W
Ulanova, Galina 35
Union Jack 27
Valois, Ninette de 13, 37
Vic-Wells Ballet 13, 37
Violin Concerto 14, 32
West Side Story 15

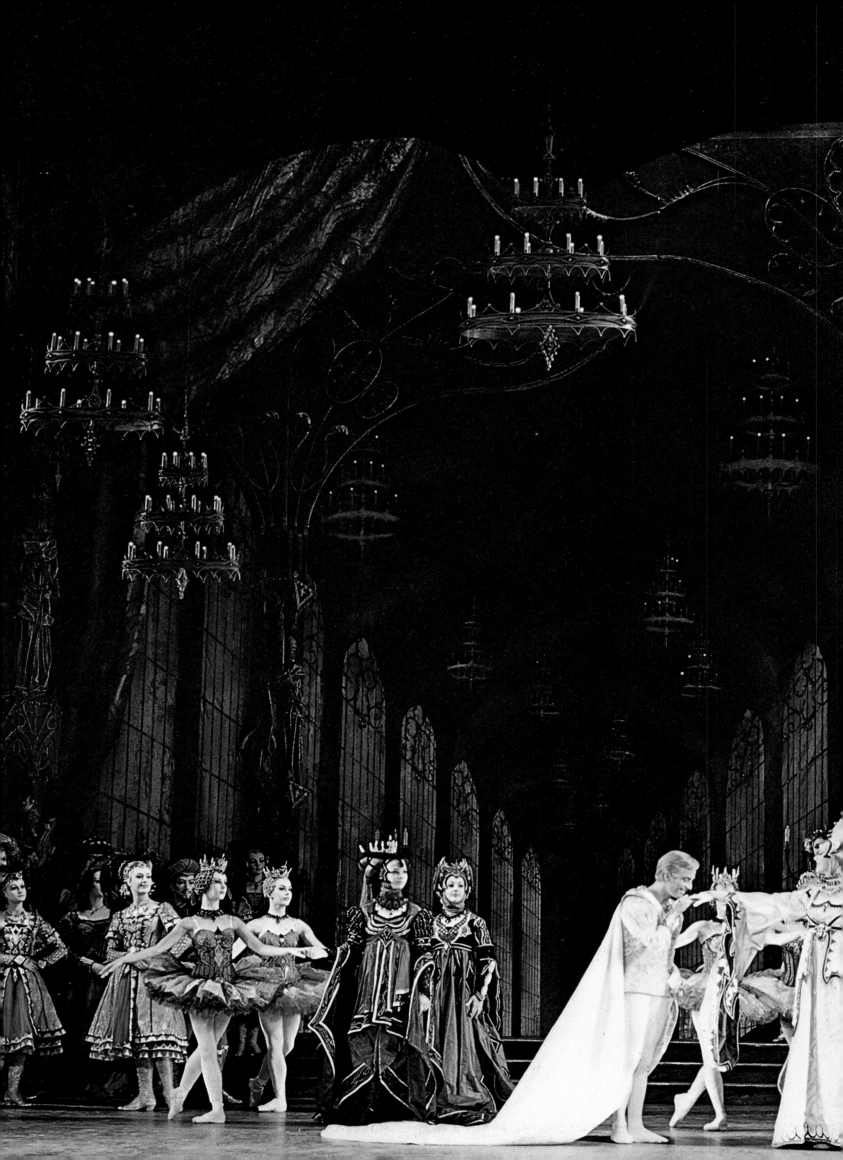